THE SH*T IS FOR REAL

tell Your Body the Good News

BY TRACEY L SCHREIBER

Cover by:

Published by:
SpeakTruth Media Group LLC
speaktruthmedia.com

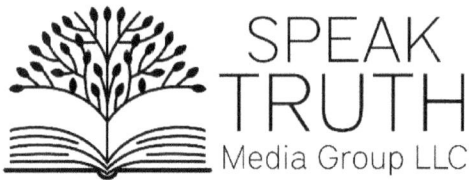

SPEAK
TRUTH
Media Group LLC

ISBN 978-1-7342646-6-1 *(pb)*

Printed in USA

Dedication

This book is dedicated to the "One."

And carrying with me the Love that there is none greater than, it is my honor to leave the safety of the ninety-nine and run to show that great Love.

Table of Contents

Foreword

Since you hold this book in your hands right now, I can tell you that the information contained within these pages will change your life forever *if* you apply what Tracey reveals. It's time for some good news! Trust me, I know your body, mind, and soul need it today!

You see, we are constantly barraged with bad news. It's no wonder our hearts feel faint within us! Once we receive negative information and allow it to take root in our hearts, our body begins to react with related physical aches and ailments. If we could make the mind, body, belief connection, we could have a joyful life filled with everything good God has planned for us.

In *The Sh*t is For Real,* Tracey masterfully lays out with life experience exactly how her physical conditions were like a lit-up Christmas tree of emotions, heartache, unforgiveness, jealousy, etc. She not only shares personal details of her victories in these areas, but the personal victories of some of the other people who encountered her and her razor-like focused intent on bringing good news into every person's life and situation.

Tracey has tapped into hidden treasure. When you learn about the wisdom she uncovered and shares in this book, you'll shake your head in disbelief saying, like her, "It was hidden in plain sight all along."

Her book will inspire and uplift you, releasing some "aha moments" in your life as you make the connection necessary to rid yourself of the negative emotions that spill over into bodily dis-ease. It's your time now to live the life you were created to live, full of blessings and good news!

Charlana Kelly
TV & Radio Host

Introduction

Well, I have finally gone and done it! I am sure it was unavoidable, *swearing* for all the world to read. For a long time, I have had a picture in my mind of my relationship with God. It is a picture of God's outstretched hand on my head, and I am swinging! When I began writing this book, the title had just one meaning. And among other things, the recent interest and craze over toilet paper and pandemics, now it can represent multiple meanings. The title is entirely obnoxious and rude, but as provocative as it is, it's an absolute labor of love. And well, a handful from birth and feisty in the Lord, I feel tailor-made for this calling! This book is intended to explore the miracles of emotional release and its practical use for healing in our bodies. I had personally prayed and seen flesh healed right before my eyes no less than three times, which was undeniably amazing in my mind. But even so, I think the fact that we can choose to give our stress to God, willingly exchange it for the positive of that emotion, and see immediate results in our bodies, is downright incredible. To think that we could choose to be in touch with firsthand miracles, time and time again. It's what I live for every day of my life! When first learning about these techniques, I couldn't get enough. Hungry for more information on the connection between our emotional and physical health, I applied what I learned and witnessed the results! It blew my mind again and again! God made us so miraculous!

I have seen far too many afflicted with chronic illness and autoimmune disease. I can remember a time when the word "autoimmune" was foreign to everyone, but it's as common as a cold these days. I have overcome all autoimmune disease and chronic illness, diagnosed, and predisposed to, and not intentionally. But by giving my emotions to God and replacing them on a very regular basis with healing thoughts and words for aches, pains, colds, and plenty of light afflictions, I have seen evidence of more significant illnesses getting headed off at the pass as a result.

For most of my life, I have been a transformation junkie. In design, dog behavior, health, and relationship. Seeing that change in everything is my passion. Like, I feel the whole world is my transformation playground. To say that strategizing and problem solving are in my blood may be a little much, but it is the absolute truth. Have you ever known someone that couldn't stop trying to figure everything out? That would be me. I analyze non-stop and see patterns in life; in Scripture, you name it. If there is a possible pattern or algorithm, I am all about it. There is a certainty in my soul that I have driven no less than thirty-five friends and family members crazy with my brain, and maybe even more than that! But I have learned not to apologize for it! God gives us our brains in all their complexities. Through the years, the unusual and extraordinary attributes of the mind have so fascinated me. The uniqueness that we all come into this world with is something I treasure. Getting to know the stories of those I meet is one of the most beautiful collections of memories I have obtained over the years.

I want to take my hunger for problem-solving and use it for the greater good and God's glory!

In this book, I want to address this autoimmune disease like the devil that it is and kick its existence right off the planet. Letting go of the emotions that cause autoimmune is something that seems to be darn near impossible for people to master. Until now! And, in light of the recent historical events of a viral pandemic, my target has widened on an epic level!

In this book, I am going to convince, empower, advertise all that emotional release and casting your cares on God, can do for a person. I want to show you in the easiest way possible. Then, get ready to hear the Good News of how a health revolution has started, and chronic "dis-ease" is kicked off the face and body of humanity! It is time to make GOOD NEWS go viral!!!

Chapter 1

Hidden in Plain Sight

"I began to see emotions in a new way;
that they are not just what we are feeling."

In 2015 my family had one intense year. Our home flooded a couple of times. The rebuilding was rough, as my husband and I stayed in our house, and our kids moved in with their grandparents not far away. I resigned from a job when I already knew I was about to get fired. It was a job where I worked as many as one hundred hours a week to compensate for understaffing. My self-esteem exposed and assaulted daily was up and down like the NASDAQ, due to my feelings of inadequacy. That year I was given a diagnosis of an underactive thyroid and my lab work noted a couple of occurrences of Epstein Barr. Several things happened towards the end of the year that changed the way I began to think about my health and life. The change was altering my thought processes on many levels.

It was after all of this that I began my journey to train as an instructor in Aromatherapy. One of the courses taught in the intensive is a modality called Emotional Release. I had never heard of it but was fascinated right from the start. Though the other subjects were interesting, I was captivated by this one and the notion that we could choose to let go of our negative emotions. And not only let go of them but replace them with a positive affirmation that would manifest healing in our bodies. At the time, I was also exploring deeper into dog behavior, learning that animals are also affected by our thoughts and emotions. I began to see emotions in a new way; that they are not just what we are feeling. They are creative on a molecular level and impact our health in ways I never imagined, which I believed right away by faith. It wasn't until a few years in that I began to grasp the science behind it. This notion of grabbing the invisible and making it tangible was thrilling and empowering! STRESS, it has been called for years. STRESS staring me in the face like an invisible foe. Never understanding the importance of letting go of stress, but also seeing how God's grace led me to forgive, which included forgiving myself! I knew it back then. Forgiveness saved my life, and really was a springboard to so much of what I needed to release. The new information about emotional release made me feel like it was "game on" to go to the next level in my life and health!

So, when I began to apply the knowledge that I learned in my journey to become an instructor, I began to see my health change. Have you ever wished that you could travel back in time and change things for a better outcome? I feel like I am rewriting my past. Now, an ailment does not come on my body that I do not look up its emotional root. Funny, but I am pretty much known as "look it up" girl. I can remember the day that I moved about twelve-hundred pounds of rock out of the clay in my friend's backyard. I thought to myself, "I have never been this strong in my life!" Now, don't get me wrong, I'm not trying to do this heavy lifting all the time, but I can. How incredible is that?

At the time, I was about to turn fifty! What was different in my life? I had avoided pre-diabetes in my earlier years, and I had been on the verge of high blood pressure as well. These afflictions got derailed by good nutrition. Some serious arthritis pain was also squashed by healthy eating. But these other ailments were new on the scene and not helped by loads of the right food. I now know that it had to do with the change in how I dealt with the emotional stress in my life! Life before this revelation had been a virtual roller coaster of stress. Did I mention that I HATE roller coasters? LOL, not Lol!

Chapter 2

A Beautiful Mess

"We are about to walk through our valleys of emotional death as we start to bring transformation to them."

In 1993 I began seeing a psychiatrist. Our life always in turmoil and anxiety; I was having the worst feelings of panic and something that felt like an elevator dropping all the time. My husband and I were a mess, and so were our finances, our home, our cars, and even our boys were the sweetest little messes. My daughter Savannah would not pop onto the scene until 1995. But you get the idea; everything was a mess!!! When I decided to seek the help of a professional, I believed that we could start to untangle that mess, so I took myself to the doctor/therapist. And then I took Ron, my husband. One of the funniest doctor's visits was when my husband went to the "headshrinker," as he called it. His doctor happened to be my doctor's husband, and she let me know my husband stared at her husband for about 45 minutes. A costly staring contest, but it gave us quite the laugh. So, I decided that I would have to figure out what the heck was wrong with me, and that might just fix us all. My first diagnosis was bi-polar.

Medicine was prescribed, then the second diagnosis of ADHD. The funny thing about these diagnoses' is that they make up two of the components of the four that are Tourette's Syndrome. My boys were both diagnosed with this a few years later. Tourette's is a real bag of fun and tricks when it comes to psychiatric issues. If you suffer from the rarest form of Tourette's that consists of Coprolalia, it's something else! Sounds like fun, right? Like a LaLaPalooza or something. But no, it is no fun! It is the part of Tourette's that gets the good laughs on late-night television. Vocalizations, involuntary cursing, or animal noises. It's a real hoot! Not!

Struggling with a throat-clearing tick most of my childhood and young adult life, coughing to clear my throat of a "phlegm-like" sensation, is what I disguised as a "sneeze" in high school. My mom even took me as a child to get my sinuses drained; it was so bad. As far as the coughing up phlegm sound, there was one class, in particular, that stressed me beyond all others. The teacher was so abrasive and challenging; it made me BIG time nervous! I could not help but "fake-sneeze" repeatedly. One night I dreamt that this teacher confided in me. He told me that he was not mean but acting that way to keep his class under control. In the dream, he told me, "I shouldn't worry." The funny thing about that dream, after I had it, I never coughed again in his class. The dream altered my thoughts and emotions, which in turn changed the stress that caused the throat-clearing ticks! Amazing!

One last note about Tourette's, the medications for the condition are so much worse than even young children blurting out swear words in the middle of church! But the thought that medication will help makes a young mom and dad turn to it to get some kind of relief,

When I tell you that I know what it is to move from glory to glory and really, it felt more like "gory to glory," I do. Don't get me wrong; we had many truly amazing times when the kids were little. It was not all bad. In fact, our life was totally nuts and beautiful at the same time. I was healed and was able to get off all medications at one awesome point in my life. And my boys, except for an "occasional" well placed swear word, are symptom-free! But when we were a young family, seriously, it was confusion and chaos a great deal of the time. Back then, we spent a lot of time managing. Survival was the goal. We always dreamt of thriving, but surviving is where we landed. I am not discounting the stretching and growing that we did. Often, we realized how the hand of God was in our life. And looking back, I should have thanked the Lord every day that we all made it to another day. Recently while driving down the road, I came up with what I thought would be a great children's song, which would have been great to sing when mine were little. It could have been our family anthem! Bear with me a moment and read these lyrics;

When everything is going right
And it's super-duper out-of-sight
I wanna praise You morning, noon, and night
And oh, I love You, Lord!
When everything is going wrong
I don't wanna even sing a song

But I shoulda known all along

I NEED TO PRAISE YOU EVEN MORE!!!

As simply *sing-songy* and straightforward as that is, it is the TRUTH!!!

So, I understand this is not easy to do. On many occasions, I gave praise and thanksgiving out of sheer desperation and then only as a token. I did not feel it whatsoever. But the words still had power. I believe this is the same in the practice of emotional release. Your pain is real! As the title of this book, the sh*t is for real! But guess what? The answer is real too! Tell your body the Good News! We are going on an adventure in this book. We are about to walk through our valleys of emotional death as we start to bring transformation to them.

Scripturally, the Lord says that He walks us through the shadow of the Valley of Death. What is the shadow? My thought is that He walks us through the "negative emotions" of the valley of death. WOW! He makes me lay down in green pastures to REST. Instead of thinking about Psalm 23, like a funeral recitation, what if we made it our picture of stress relief for the living? What if we got a vision of that valley blooming after we walk through it with the Lord? Like, not just surviving our circumstances but transforming them, there it is! Transformation! That is the kind of thing I cannot get enough of in my life! Your body needs to hear the Good News!!! Try this next exercise out the next time you start to feel stressed by whatever is going on in your life.

Ok, if you, by chance right now, have a headache or maybe even a backache, heck any pain, I want you to do this. Close your eyes, and imagine that the pain has a color. My stepmom, Laura, told me about this method a few years ago. Do it! If you have never done this, it might seem crazy. But go ahead, give the pain a color. Now hold your hands up and make a circle and give your pain a size, now pause and see how you feel. If your pain is not gone, give it another try, do it until the pain is gone.

Now how do you feel? If you did this and your pain was stress-related, you may just be feeling total relief or be well on your way to feeling relief. I have used this technique primarily when I get one of those headaches that happen after pushing myself to finish something at a client's house. I love to be able to vacate before family members make it back home at the end of the day so they can have their beautiful home back. A desire that has, on many occasions, landed me with a nagging headache. I have used the method for shoulder pain as well, and it worked in an instant. So, if you had a headache or pain and it is gone, YAY!!! What you did is take the controls of your body. God made us so miraculous. He created our bodies to function with an advantage over certain death. Your pain could be distracting your mind from stress, or your pain could be pointing to your stress.

A little bit of stress is good. Like if you need to run from the bear, which oddly enough, I have done in real life. Long summer camp story! Lol! The emotion that gives your body the signal and power to move is vital. But stress that is chronic or unproductive is harmful and must be avoided or alleviated. So, your brain will distract you from your stress by giving you pain. But essentially, you just called out the stress, gave it color and size, and your brain told it to go you do not need it. Kind of like punching your stress pain in the face and sending it packing! I believe this is very much like when we use emotional release for our health. We pin-point that unhealthy feeling and call it out. When we choose to give our hurt, anger, procrastination, or any of the myriad of stressful emotions that we feel, to God, we will see results! But just giving it to God and letting it go is not enough.

We need to tell our bodies the Good News. I say Jesus went to all that trouble for us; you know the story, the greatest LOVE STORY EVER!!! So, tell it to your body! Because of that great love story, we can have story time with our bodies. Making this real in your mind and legitimizing it is the key. You have not because you ask not, which is totally scriptural. And I like to think you have not because you *command* not! If your headache went away by giving it a size, a color, and a name, you might not believe the rest of this book is necessary. But whether you are convinced or not, my friend, read on! We are about to dismantle the hold the enemy has on our bodies.

Chapter 3

Wednesday's Child is Full of Woah!

*"Running the race with wild abandon,
blessing all that would dare to get in your way!"*

I was born on Wednesday. Thinking about that poem and the whole of Wednesday's child is full of woe; it could not have been truer on many days of the first half of my life. Tell me if any of this sound familiar:

Pain

Woe

Martyr

Anger

Bitter

Control

Victim

Wounded

Ashamed

Jealousy!!!

"JeaLOUSY" (my lousy greatest battle) is cured with thankfulness! My Self-talk on gratitude as a weapon against jealousy will come a bit later. Talk about a "ME TOO" movement. How many of us have not been exposed to some sort of abuse as kids? I can remember sitting in my middle school, so full of emotions, and wanting to be liked and loved. And then, at the beginning of one of my classes, my best friend dumps me as she tells me I am not popular enough to be her friend. This all for my classmates to hear. TERRIBLE! The most telling thing about her words as I look back is that they were what I already felt about myself. When I tell you, little people-pleasing Tracey was devastated. Sadly, this moment would be a defining moment and something I would need to give to God years later. The friend did make amends with me after quite a bit of time. And shortly after she terminated our friendship in middle school, God sent me another fantastic friend! But the message that her words sent to me on a molecular level stuck with me for a very long time. I know now also that God used that rejection to send me in another direction. Though we made amends, we did not continue as active friends. Some of the greatest and most sudden rejections I have now come to believe to be the hand of God.

So, now when I think about how the world is and the kind of person I want to be in it, I have to confess the "Wednesday's Child full of WOAH!!!" is what comes to my mind. Changing my perspective and who I am in the story of my life, I can now say I have gone *from woe to Woah*! People are hungry for the WOAH!!! Not woe! There's a difference. *Woah* is an awestruck wonder and surprise. It's good. *Woe* is sorrow or distress. Did you catch that? Di-stress! Woe puts stress on you. Woah relieves it.

I love waking up in the morning and thinking about the tremendous possibilities of the day. Did you know that you can change the course of a person's day by spreading a little cheer? It doesn't even take a lot of it. Good news goes a long way! And sometimes, it is just taking the time to look up from what you're focused on and smile at someone. I have always wanted to be able to do Parkour! Talk about a WOAH-type of activity! Don't know what Parkour is? Well, it's an activity where someone quickly runs through an area, negotiating obstacles by running, jumping, and climbing. I watch with amazement at the seemingly limitless abilities of those renegade athletes! I hated gymnastics as a child, but something about watching Parkour that seems so freeing! When I think about running the race of life and moving with God through it, it kind of reminds me of their free limitless movements. Running the race with wild abandon, blessing all that would dare to get in your way! And then bonus, grab a hand and invite them to run with you!!! Maybe this is why I am so passionate about people getting free from the constraints of illness! I will say it, probably more than once in this book, but I just want to yell it here as I run towards "the good" in life, "Take up your sickbed and walk!" Or better yet, "Take up your sickbed and run!" WOAH!!!

Chapter 4

Tell Your Body the Good News!

"We can preach the Good News to the 37.2 trillion cells in our body."

It makes me think of going into all the world, preaching, and telling everyone the Good News. Recently I saw a tribute to Reinhart Bonnke, the German-born evangelist, who has ministered the Gospel to millions at a time. If you ever need to see a compelling picture of millions coming together for a greater good in one accord, you need to look up a Bonnke crusade video on YouTube. When I look at his videos, they give me a picture of GOOD winning. I thought, though, when I saw Evangelist Bonnke and those millions of sweet souls in Nigeria, about how many cells are in our bodies, which is a great visual! Then it occurred to me. We can preach the Good News to the millions of cells in our body! Breathing, moving, existing creates free radicals in your body. The science behind the process is best described as because we live, we die! Plants go in and infuse the oxidative stress with antioxidants. Emotion messenger molecules can be flushed out, but we need to be filled with positive information to replace the negative message that was sent. So, like Bonnke, we can be our own evangelist to our millions of cells in our bodies. A prayer that I love to pray is,

"Lord heal my unbelief." There is a Bible verse that talks about this, and it's so incredible to me (Mark 9:23). A father's son was vexed with all manner of "unclean spirits." When he went to Jesus, the Lord said, "Only believe, all things are possible to them that believe." The father replied to Jesus, "Help me with my unbelief." And, his little boy was healed.

Negative emotions? If you believe ALL things, not just good things are possible. Mark 9:23 is a Scripture that I have spent the most time pondering, meditating on, and mulling over! My thoughts (I call them my "believer.") and attitude and emotions need healing daily. Heck on an hourly basis! When my "believer" is broken, that is when I ask God to heal it. I choose to speak what I want to see! And I am not talking about "Jeanie in a bottle" stuff here. In faith, I begin to talk it out with God. The funny thing about emotional release is that for me, most of the time, it is quite emotionless. At least until about thirty seconds later, when the ache or pain is gone. Then I am jumping up and down, celebrating how miraculous God made us. Did I say that already? God made us so miraculous! There have been a few times that the healing was not instant, but the improvement began right away. Recently I started to go next level on the emotional release in my abdomen area. As I said earlier, in so many words, this issue is my ground zero for sure. I wanted to get the six-pack abs that I never had, even when I was young. So about five days into my next level ab work, I strained a muscle. I watched a video online to make sure I was doing it right so that I wouldn't injure myself. When the very sharp pain happened, the first thought I had was, "Oh crap, I must be doing this wrong." I continued with a few more reps and realized that I needed to ease up for that morning.

Later I had a thought to look and see what the alarm point was for the area. Hey, what a concept! I looked it up, and the alarm point in my ab area muscle pain was called the adrenal cortex. The emotions that have to do with this area are feelings of being defenseless, aggression, and fear of confrontation. I immediately realized this is a list of emotions that the dogs at the shelter where I volunteer can feel. Aggression, not so much, but you get the idea! So, I gave it all to God and then replaced them all verbally with the positive outlook emotions. Even though the pain didn't disappear entirely till 24 hours later, I thought that was amazing, considering I thought I had torn a muscle!

Living in the present is a fine art. Cesar Millan says it all the time. You cannot live in the past or anticipate the future when it comes to working with troubled dogs. The Bible discusses fear and worries at length. When it asks the question, "Can anyone of you, by worrying, add a single hour to your life?" (Matthew 6:27). I say heck no to that! As a matter of fact, it could do just the opposite! Living in the moment is really a fine art and practice that does worlds of good for your body. It is what everyone is talking about, being present. Without a doubt, there is enough science and data to prove it. But just because we know the science of something doesn't mean that we will apply it, necessarily. Scripture tells us that worrying in advance does us no good. In my work with dogs, I marvel at how they pick up on our thoughts and the related emotions. Your family dog can be a good indication of how you feel. Sometimes they are a mirror, reflective of this. The nervousness, anxiety, anger, and being preoccupied with negative thoughts. That's it! What is occupying your mind? And how is it affecting your body? Occupy!!! That is where we take ground in our health. Tell your body the Good News! Heal your unbelief. Jesus did the work. We must hand our stress to Him. I get it. Boy, do I get it! It may seem impossible. If you are suffering from an autoimmune disease or any illness chronic or not, the way to give it up may seem illusive. But like forgiveness, that we are commanded to do, we begin to speak these things away. Talk about Freedom of Speech! Tell your body the Good News! We choose it! And this is not anything new. But why is it so difficult and seemingly painful to let it go? Over the Christmas holiday, the local Christian radio station played an inspirational commercial of sorts saying something clever about hope, "When I lose IT, I choose IT." Why is it that good advice can always be put in a poem? I guess it's kind of like a modern-day Psalm! Sing your body the Good News!!!

Come on; this is a battle! I once told a dear friend of mine who was battling cancer, that we needed to throw everything at it! This girl is one of the top five most amazing women I have the blessing of knowing. Her attitude is pure love and sunshine! She chose prayer, chemo, oils, nutrition, emotional release to kick that crap to the curb. I told her of a beetle that I heard about that folks said could eradicate cancer from your body. One day I investigated it on Google, and there was an article that stated this beetle emitted a chemical in your body that would kill cancer. People reported that they put the live bugs in capsules and took them internally! I told her we would order the bugs!!!

Illness of any kind is a battle! And really, that is the truth when it comes to any type of obstacle, and ultimately the battle is God's! Cast your cares on Him as commanded in Scripture. Why do we not take that one as seriously as the command to forgive? Is it because that is where we give ourselves a break? We have value! Give yourself a break and tell your body the Good News!

Forbidding yourself to give what is troubling and stressing you out to God is something that I have observed again and again. It is because I am always trying to talk people out of being sick and sad. And those that suffer from these sinister ailments damn near refuse to give it to God—just saying! Let it go! It has no purpose for your LIFE! What if I told you on the other side of letting go of those emotions, and keeping at it for continued health, you could avoid surgery, lose weight, run faster, ENJOY LIFE more! Leaving the all too familiar land called *Victim* and move into the land of *Giant Slayer*! In the next chapter, I am going to tell you a story about a woman who paints one heck of a before and after picture of what I'm encouraging you to do here. And let's see if that sparks something!

Chapter 5

And the Emmy Goes To

"I had a moment when I decided to put on a new wardrobe."

She always wondered, even from a very young age, if she mattered. It wasn't that her parents never made her feel loved and cared for because they absolutely did both. But she longed for a great deal of positive feedback and acceptance beyond the norm. Can a child be born with a people-pleasing habit? She loved absorbing grownup conversations and wanted to be in on them from a young age. She got along with children her age, but it seemed that she always desired more. "Notice me, notice me," was the dialogue that played over and over in her mind. And though her attention span was racing all the time, she was as bright as a button. She would not realize this until years later. But as a child, she pretended all things. No one would have ever known about all that she carried in her heart. Pretending was her talent. All those smarts got pushed to the wayside so that she could cope. Looking normal was her way of survival when all was not. So, as she grew, she began to major on people-pleasing.

Fast forward to her adult life. Imagine a woman sitting on a pile of trash in the worst part of town, digging through garbage in the middle of the night when questionable characters walked the city streets. There she would be. Was this woman crazy? Sometimes night after night, she went out looking for something she could save and make beautiful again. Her husband was at a loss as to how he could stop her. She was the conductor, of all the madness, in a wildly out-of-control life.

It was never "why me?" that she asked. It was a no brainer. Her thoughts were always, "Of course me!" "Victim" was her designer label and the wardrobe she quietly wore every day. "Anger and "control" were the loud accessories and "shame" her undergarments. These were the clothes that she wore, day in and day out until she didn't. Her life was so dramatic, like daytime drama-ish, but the truth! And there's no cliff-hanger here; this woman in the story was me until she wasn't!

I had a moment when I decided to put on a new wardrobe. I decided I needed that outfit you get when you choose to make Jesus your new EVERYTHING! I know there were times when I checked the receiving Christ thing off my list. Like I said, the words when they were just a token. And then, one day, I decided to go all-in and choose Him for real and then choose to let Him remodel my heart. It was the fixer-upper of fixer-uppers. It was, without a doubt, a defining moment in my life and the real beginning of becoming completely free of all those afflictions!

Ron and I saw miracle after miracle. I can remember the time I had heard a pastor say that God seems to answer the prayers of "baby Christians" fast! I like fast! So, one day I told Ron that we needed to pray as a couple. What a concept. I told him that I heard our prayers would get answered fast, and so I asked him what he would like to pray for right then. He thought for a second, and then he said, "Rain!" We had been in a drought for so long that I knew we would know all of this was true if we got rain. So, we held hands, and I prayed for rain. We agreed with an Amen, and then in a moment, I had a burst of excitement, did what I call my little excitement fists shaking thing in front of me, and exclaimed, "Wouldn't it be awesome if tomorrow there were thunderstorms all around?" The following day as we were driving home, we were trying to call each other from our cars on our flip phones. When we finally got in touch, we were both excitedly trying to find out if the other one saw the lightning and thunder surrounding our area. He told me there was rain in the parking lot of his job, and I told him it was beginning to shower a bit at our house! At that moment, we both knew that praying together was the key to our future. Our first prayer as a couple, and it was answered the next day! And quite specifically, the words I spoke out in an excited, childlike way with childlike gestures came to pass! Now answered prayer had occurred too many times to count. I have, over the years, had several dear friends tell me I am a prophet and don't even know it. I would always tell them they were crazy and that when I think of a prophet, I get this Bible guy imagery wearing crazy clothes and all. Usually, I look down at my outfit with paint or spackle on it and say, "Hmm!" I have noticed words coming to pass when I am so excited for the answer like a little child. My granddaughter, on my birthday, made the same little gesture with her hands after I told her great things were happening this year! Which, by the way, even a worldwide

30

pandemic cannot shake me from believing. I know that when crap is hitting the fan, God's GRACE is hitting that fan in a significant way!!!

So, in all of the pain from my childhood, real or imagined, the enemy was never able to touch my childlike faith. The ability to jump back up and believe to the point that it just seems ridiculous and stupid is something that I have gotten really good at and have been able to take that childlike excited hope-filled gesture and punch the devil square in the face!

Chapter 6

Go Ahead Be Childish

"I have found in years where I was my most-brattiest self in the Lord; I had never felt more loved!"

Like the faith of a little child, Jesus talked about in Matthew 18:2—4. Childish, I don't want to be childish; I want to be the most CHILDEST I can be. That is the thing! When we have the faith of a little child, we believe we can do anything. Turning fifty-one, I have come to think about anti-aging more than ever! I actually do feel stronger than when I was fifteen! Even so, I continue to search, as do many, for the fountain of youth. At one point, I did a trial of singing worship to improve my skin. And in the video, I believed I saw my skin transform right before my eyes! I know, so strange. Now iPhones ARE deceptively awesome at transforming how we look on selfie-mode, but Worship Therapy, now that is what I am talking about for reversing the aging process!!! In fact, the Greek word for worship is "*therapeuo,*" like therapy! Do you see a theme here? God is the Source! Not the bad-ass mother load, I recently read someone say, but God almighty. HE made us so miraculous! And what Jesus did for us on the Cross made it permanent. In a Bible verse, Jesus said, "let the little children come." He didn't give them a list of instructions. He simply stated to let them come. Children naturally gravitate toward peace, pure love, and stability. These are the things that Jesus inherently was and is. Very young children don't spend time strategizing to get to what they want. They simply move forward and go to what they are drawn to naturally. It was when I watched my sweet grandson, Maverick, recently learning to walk that I realized they have no fear. It took only a few times of falling on his journey to walking that he learned to be guarded. I want to always run toward the destiny God has for me in perfect health, unguarded, and stress-free! Lord, heal my Un-Child!

Interestingly, we give a negative assignment to the word childish or childishness. I'm not referring to refusing to grow up like a Peter Pan-like Syndrome. But I hear time and time again from fellow believers that they feel guilty for things. They are always in pursuit of what is right, but that they feel guilty for having fallen short. Well, I have found in years where I was my most brattiest self in the Lord, I had never felt more loved! There were plenty of times when I cried out to God for situations that seemed hopeless and scary. But what I am talking about is when I pulled up my draw bridge and stuck my middle finger at the world and decided to harbor my anger. Literally doing everything, I could not let go of the things that caused my upset—all the while suffering the pain in my body from it. Even though my pain and suffering were real, I felt that I was never alone and very much loved by God. I am so thankful for the knowledge of what it means to let go of the negative.

I was in the car with my granddaughter recently, and she kept singing over and over her version of the famous song from the Disney movie, Frozen. For several days I tried to figure out what her special lyrics were. She is three, so everything she says or sings or does is so cute. But after analyzing for a good three or four days, I was amazed at what I deciphered from her words. Wet it go, Wet it go, an-a-doan-chew. She sang this over and over, and it played over and over in my mind. Then suddenly, it clicked! Of course, wet it go, wet it go, was easy to translate. Let it go, let it go, and then like a lightning bolt, the next translation, "an-a-doan-chew," and why don't you?!

Can you say out of the mouths of babes! Let it go, let it go, and why don't you? What emotions are you hanging on to right now? I believe that God sustains us until we can get to a place where we begin to choose to let it go. Me, behind my virtual and mental drawbridge, was proof of that. And truthfully, there are so many ways to do it as you begin to let it go! My personal favorite is to just simply speak that I choose to let it go and then replace it with the positive and or Scripture. You can use essential oils to affect your limbic system directly. The almost instant result I have seen time and time again is when people inhale Peppermint essential oil, and joy comes over their face! It is quite literally refreshing!

Emotional release is an powerful modality. And sometimes you must go next level in this type of approach to healing. If you are trying to release and you are not getting anywhere, there are a couple of things I have discovered of late that you can try. If there is pain in your body and the release is not coming, you can think about someone else that you may be worried about at that moment. And then think of how they are feeling and release and replace with those thoughts in mind. On several occasions, I have had to think about this. And when I thought about lifting up the emotions, I felt as though they were feeling; I got immediate relief! Sometimes we will carry a friend or a loved one's pain. I am a pro at that, understanding I could feel sorry for a pinecone. That is a longstanding joke between Bev and me about my "hyper-empathy"!

Let me diverge for a moment and tell you about my bestie Bev. Enter Beverly Carter. My fantastic friend for years, confidant, instructor, mentor, and accomplice. She has had more to do with growing my confidence in my gifts and talents than I can write in one book. Bev likes to call me her memory, and I am happy to remind her of all the blessings she has been and done so easily, but readily forgets. It almost seems like a type of "humility amnesia" or something! When one day you're chatting over coffee and find out that you and your best friend have taken in the same homeless lady and her son, it leads you to believe that you have twin powers or something for good, of course, LOL! Bev is a treasure. Now back to my hyper-empathy.

Another trick up my sleeve is to take the concept of giving your pain a size and a color that I mentioned in an earlier chapter and put it on paper! Like art therapy! Draw it! Color it! You can write it out or illustrate it out!! As an artist, this is something I can totally relate to in my gift and life. When I was younger, I met a family that, with art therapy, overcame a significant loss and tragedy. The children painted their way to freedom. To me, it was so powerful. You could see the progression of their healing in their pictures. It is all a part of telling your body the good news. Let it go and end up with a beautiful masterpiece of health! You can use tapping: which is so simple but can be highly effective in releasing trauma. EFT Emotional Freedom Technique is another way to find relief. That old commercial for V-8, you know the one where the people in the commercial smack their forehead with a burst of surprise and say, "I should've had a V-8!" There it is! The aha moment! A big TAP! When working at the animal shelter with dogs that have been through an unbelievable amount of trauma, I love to use Lavender oil and tap on their hip areas to release the tension. The great thing about dogs is that you can see them begin to release their trauma and go on to live in the present and thrive! Which is very much like little children, too! Why can't we do that same thing as easily? I have learned so much from becoming a grandmother and also in this work at the animal shelter. New Rules for myself: The dog poops, I can poop. The dog can let it go; I can let it go. Little children and puppies' default are love and joy; my default is love and joy. YAY!!! I choose; it's that simple!

Chapter 7

Provocative with Purpose

"the sudden results that I have seen in my health through emotional release is nothing short of addicting."

So, it is a long and well-known fact that a hug, a massage, and even exercise can cause emotional outbursts. There is also this thing that I do that I just absolutely hate. Something will make me laugh so hard I cry and not just cry. I will be laughing hysterically and giggling, and I can't stop! Suddenly I am overcome with hysterical crying like my feelings are hurt. As crazy as this is and as much as I hate it, I think it is like an involuntary clearing out of emotionally pent up energy. Kind of like a sneeze for my soul! Afterward, for a few hours or days, I will feel emotionally hungover.

Also, when you get your body moving, it gets your molecules moving too! Your movement begins to shake things up on a cellular level. It is always my intension when I set out to lose weight that I purpose to release fat and release and replace my negative emotions as well. When I exercise my body intensely, I do the same. I think this is just like when your body rejects cigarettes at first and then craves them. Smoking cigarettes is habit-forming; you can replace that habit with something healthy. You better know that at first, your body will want to reject the exercise, but then will crave it. On a side note, this is the same with food. We all know how addicting unhealthy food is. But I believe that raw "live" food has the same powerful effect on the good! One day a friend of mine and her daughter made an all raw food meal for another friend's birthday. She literally made a dip called ugly dip! It was some kind of ugly! But as we stood around the kitchen island and ate it, we quickly devoured it all! I have to say the dip did not taste remarkable, but the next morning I woke up and thought, "I need more ugly dip!" My body knew! I think this was the same reaction as the spontaneous outburst of laughter, leading to a cry. I believe that my body is created to understand what it needs and desires. So, what if we participate with how God made us, and choose to take the emotional release to a whole new level. We endeavor to release toxic emotions for optimal health!

Nearly every day, for quite some time, I have traveled up to the local shelter in our city. The large adoptable dogs are in great need early in the morning to get taken out so they can relieve themselves. This early morning shift is one that I am working on bringing attention to as I have found out the curious and excellent benefits of working with these large dogs. Very early in the morning, I get up and begin to take care of my pack as I start my morning routine. Self-care is an area I have struggled in for years. There is something, though, about taking care of so many dogs in the morning. It causes you to realize your needs matter. The lessons I learn from dogs grows nearly every day. That is where I get my new mantra, "The dog poops, I poop!" For starters, I once used lemon myrtle for procrastination on the large intestine alarm point. Well, not to be all TMI, but the thing I procrastinate on the most is the afore-mentioned subject, pooping. Within just a few minutes, the procrastination on that was taken care of after applying the lemon myrtle essential oil. Then, bonus, I went out, painted the back deck of my house, and did two years of taxes. Lemon myrtle on the large intestine alarm point (upper abdomen) is, without a doubt, more effective than a double espresso shot, in my opinion! Here is the truth, though, in light of that information. If you have no lemon myrtle, you can still speak the words to release and replace procrastination!

By going to the shelter early in the morning and on most mornings, I'm alone and walking an average of twenty dogs; sometimes as many as thirty-five, you can work on buried emotions that surface quite readily. At one point, I asked God, "Why am I here"? I volunteered to work at the shelter to help volunteers get the best out of the dogs by offering to teach behavior techniques to new volunteers. So to better equip myself for the task, I began learning the ins and outs of the shelter by volunteering in the large dog area. While doing this, I discovered a great need at this early hour of the morning. On average, twenty to thirty dogs needed to go potty. Can I just say it here with apologies? The shit is for real!! So, when this need became apparent, I decided to fill it as much as possible. It wasn't long before I questioned my sanity and asked God that question, "Why am I here"? The answer came very quickly; a precise answer impressed on me is that God had opened a problematic door that He equipped me to walk through. Which was not exactly the WHY answer I'd hoped for, but the WHY grew increasingly apparent to me. Shelter work will naturally lead you to your own emotional work, the kind that anyone would imagine! After my first day working with these dogs, I felt every muscle in my core as a bonus! I do hard physical things regularly and never get sore. I use nutrition to overcome oxidative stress and rarely experience sore muscles from a workout. This workout at the large dog area quite frankly kicked my ass! Why was that? I am very much into going to the next level these days, and I believe the Lord is accommodating me in this. While I am working on helping this organization and filling a need, loving on dogs, and loving on employees and other volunteers, God is working on me. The area where I felt the sore muscles were in every square inch of my core. All of the alarm points for the negative emotions I struggle with are in this area. Coincidence? I think not! Check this out;

Anger- Liver

Possessive- Abdomen

Control-Stomach

Jealousy-Armpit

Exercise-Exorcism LOL

But seriously, while I am working out physically while taking care of these dogs, I am reaching new areas of stored emotions to work on as well. It is a win-win and a win!!! Transformation can come at a cost. But I am totally into optimization, and this shelter-exercise thing is for real!!! If I am going to have my ass kicked almost every morning at

6:30, I am going to help some dogs, help some people, help my physical body, and release those negative emotions to boot! I bet the devil never saw that coming!!!

I'm "Workin" *in Progress*

A funny observation that I have made through these past five years is that the more I improve, the more I want to improve. Stagnating in the "good-enough" is so not my style, nor is it for many others. And the sudden results that I have seen in my health through emotional release is nothing short of addicting. It's a good obsession! I guess we label our good obsessions as passion. LOL! How do we get to that place though, when everything looks like a no-win, dead-end, lousy livin', crummy bummer situation? Well, it is what I like to call talking yourself out of being sick and sad. As I said earlier, this is a mission of mine for others and myself! I have made myself my own living experiment due to my analyzing addiction! One experiment I will never forget is when I, on purpose, smiled myself out of a terrifying situation.

I found myself, and my good friend Bev, needing to get our kayak back to shore after realizing that our walrus watching expedition was not the right activity for us! We were on a luxurious women's retreat at a beautiful mansion on the beach in Mexico! It was terrific, and the activities were over-the-top for sure, but I am more of a shoreline, shell finding kind of girl. Paddling back, I realized that the Sea of Cortez below us was about 1000 feet deep. Suddenly, manta rays were, flying through the air around us. I was sure an enormous shark was lurking below, making its imagined existence perfect for the scene we were paddling through at that moment. Hearing somewhere that smiling makes your brain release feel-good chemicals, I felt I needed them to release in the worst way. So, as we both paddled back, I had the cheesiest grin on my face! And, good news, it helped ease my panic; whether the terror was real or not didn't matter to my brain. My smile told my brain something, and it communicated to my body. Can you stop the fight or flight mode with a smile? I have decided that our bodies need a smile *and* what it can do for us. Our bodies need to release negative emotions. If the last message sent to your body is RUN, then you need to give your body a break to release and replace it with a message that you are safe!

When you are in this fight or flight mode, a dog feels the need to protect you because of this message in your cells. The energy you are projecting is that something in you is in flight mode. The dog doesn't know why, but it knows. Check this out!

Three years ago, I decided to dig in and begin to release the negative emotion of "possessiveness." It is the very opposite of letting go! The alarm point for this negative emotion is called "abdomen" and is, in fact, on the abdomen. I think this is so interesting because my obsessive, possessive behavior started with my kids, and well, that was where they were stored for a good nine months at the beginning of their sweet lives. Now there is a healthy dose of possessiveness that is just part of motherhood. But I am talking about a very unhealthy amount. Some would have called me a helicopter mom, but in retrospect, I was like a whole fleet of helicopters! I could give you examples but will spare my kids the replay. This behavior did not end with my kids. It flowed over onto my husband, friends, pets, the property; you name it. I believe it was a massive part of my issues early on.

Have a look at your email and photos. I never delete mine and always buy more data to store it all. I am not saying that this is a sure sign, but it has seemed that I want to hold on to it all. When I started attacking this possessiveness and working on releasing and replacing, it appears that my abdomen started shaping up and flattening out. For years my mom would tell me, "Suck it in, Tra!" Moms, you gotta love em, Lol! Suck it in. Funny, but that is what I was doing emotionally and literally like a human vortex of control.

No one could escape! I was basically hoarding life but not just my own, my family, and friends as well. So, as I began to punch this possessiveness in the gut (abdomen), I began to get a knot in my throat! Well, of course, one day, while working on an up and coming book together, I told my good friend Bev my symptom. We looked it up the "laryngeal prominence," aka the knot in my throat was the negative emotion, possessiveness. I was like, "Are you kidding me?" and Bev was like, "Nope!" I had the knot in my throat for over two weeks.

I began to release and replace and, funnily enough, ended up having my own come to Jesus moment, even with my book writing. For years I had worked on getting my books written and published. As I looked at my countless attempts, I realized it was one big train wreck! I had been trying to do all of it in my own strength. My last name

Schreiber actually, means "writer, " in German it means pencil pusher! So, I am just a scribe. A later revelation hit me about my name as I began writing this book, but I am saving that story for the end. So, when I saw that I needed to let my sweet friend author her book and support her as a friend instead of co-author, it led me that day to do one of the most incredible acts to release the possessiveness that I have done thus far. I stood on top of my bed, sorry mom, and made a declaration out loud, saying, "I'm handing over my writing and my attempts at writing past and present to God."

I even gave my name Schreiber, the pencil pusher, to God. When I talk to my ceiling, I am talking to God. You would not believe the conversations I have had with God through the sheetrock. That is actual proof that God loves me and puts up with all of my shenanigans! And on a side note, God understands my great desire to possess the land. I mean, He commanded us to go in and take the land, and I am the girl that will run to be the first to stick the flag in the ground! But I gave it all to Him and told Him to give me back what He wanted me to have. I know we cannot boss the Lord around, but it was a heartfelt surrender of all that I was trying to possess in this area. And it wasn't just anything I handed over. It was and is something I have felt I am born to do.

Writing has always seemed to be the land calling my name. The next day as I stood in my studio waiting to leave for my husband's visit to the eye doctor, one of the books I'd planned to write flooded into my head. And at that moment, I stopped my brain and said, "Brain, stop it! We have not heard from God on the matter! And brain, you are just trying to write the book in my head instead of on the computer!" I know, who the heck talks to their brain? Within fifteen minutes of that declarative moment, on the way to our appointment, my now publisher called me saying she had been thinking about my children's book, and she wanted to help me make that book a reality! "What?!" Could this be happening? To me, this was a straight-up, clear-cut, beyond awesome miracle! Not only is God healing your body when you give negative, unhealthy emotions to Him, He will also bring your dreams to pass in the process! He turned my "possessive" into possessing the land and all that is given to us by God. Thankful, thankful, thankful!!! Did I mention that I am so thankful? I will say now I joyfully spend time in my studio working on writing and illustrating. God is so Good!

Chapter 8

There's No Such Thing as Self-Checkout

"We are made to laugh!"

"There is no such thing as self-checkout!" A little something I say every time I am going through the self check-out line at the store. I say things like, "Hey, look, there's a camera on me! I have always wanted my own television show!" Or this, "Wow! The more I buy, the harder I have to work!" How about this one? My idea of self-checkout is where I look in the mirror and say, "Girl, you look good today!" Or even something like, "Maybe this is all an evil plot to get me to order online and have my stuff delivered, so they never have to put up with my amateur joke collection again!" Yes, these are jokes. A comedy routine that I know my adult children are so glad they get to miss and that my grandchildren love entirely. Because, well, let's face it, they love everything I do! But seriously, do you have a regimen of laughter? In this terribly funny, unfunny world we live in, you need one! My husband and I owe the survival of our marriage to God almighty and His invention of laughter!

I have worked on collecting material for a comedy routine for years. I know the time I took up the violin at forty, it probably seemed like the biggest joke ever! But it wasn't. I practiced obsessively many hours a day for several years. I can play "Twinkle, Twinkle, Little Star" like a total rock star, but beyond that, I am not sure you could even recognize my other songs. When my parents let me know that they didn't hear an actual song in my extravagant stylings, I decided that I did not appreciate the honesty! The next time they asked why they hadn't heard me play for the longest time, I promptly let them know that they would have to buy tickets!

In all honesty, I picked that violin up and started playing to keep the arthritic onslaught of my fingers at bay. But I discovered other advantages to my new-found obsession. Though I never became great at playing, I could strategically use my practice time as a bargaining tool when my kids were teenagers. If you don't clean your room, I will practice, practice, practice! It has provided me with comedy material for years. Here is my point; laughter is medicine. It is healing. Even the laughter that sends you into hysterical crying. I believe laughter is an amazing doorway into emotional release. Find ways to laugh. For some, this will be an effortless assignment. For others, it will be impossible but do it anyway. I believe the more you laugh, the more you will want to laugh. Here is some science to grab hold of right now. When we laugh, our bodies release feel-good chemicals! With that information, it should also cause you to want to laugh and make others laugh as well. Go into all the world preaching and teaching people to love and laugh!!! It can overshadow the bitter and ugly that emotionally are the roots of viral infections!

How do you like those apples! Get off your Apple and plug into the beautiful and good! My mom has told me for years that as a tiny baby, I would laugh and laugh! Also, I can remember how I could find a piece of fuzz and turn it into a spider on a thread, and make it move around as if alive, completely cracking myself up! I recently noticed a little boy in the Walmart return line doing the same thing. He didn't have an iPhone to amuse him, he had an old school piece of string dancing it around like a spider. He, too, was cracking up, and as he did, his mom was on her phone, totally unaware. My point is we are made to laugh! If a tiny infant can laugh, I think laughter could be our default if we choose it! Here is an assignment for healing; turn off all news, real, fake, and otherwise. Talk about TMI! Reign in what your mind is exposed to daily and give yourself a break. The repeated onslaught of negativity is like an overdose of toxins. Then exchange all of that for laughter, which is a healthy habit you can form. Suggestion: Addicting and refreshing, viral videos, a baby's laughter is better than any comedy routine!

Try this exercise, write down five hilarious memories from your childhood. Another healthy brain assignment: Spend time meditating on those good, carefree, joy-filled memories. I use these memories as a reset button. I can remember things from childhood back to a very young age. One time my dad told me he could remember chasing ducks as a toddler. Remember back when you felt pure joy and spend time thinking about it, a time when STRESS was not in your vocabulary. If you had a childhood that didn't allow for happiness, I am so sorry. It seems that this is not an uncommon situation. But I want you to do this exercise, as I believe this is more important for you. Sit back and close your eyes and begin to see yourself as a child and begin to imagine the happiness and laughter that you did not have—first giving your unhappy memories to God. Then in your mind, envision that situation going in the direction of happy, fulfilled, and loved. Your brain will begin to see it as the new reality. We can't change the past, but in our mind and body, we can imagine it differently. And that will begin to change how we live now! Re-imagining your childhood! Talk about a neighborhood of make-believe that could change your life! It is the kind of self-checkout I am talking about right here!

Chapter 9

What's Your Poison?

"Perspective is a powerful cocktail that we give our brain."

A question I remember asking my dad years ago was, "Dad, can the devil physically hurt us?" I remember him telling me that he could not lay a finger on us in the natural realm. I have never really liked the book of Job for light reading, and it seems at first glance, it contradicts my dad's perspective. But there's a verse that is quoted quite often that I want to look at further. "The thing I have feared the most has…" I can't even bring myself to write the full sentence! Fear is talked about almost synonymously with stress. Putting stress in place of fear in that verse, well, you get the idea. Even as I write this, I am in the middle of believing the flu away for my husband. Yesterday, he called me with the news that out on his delivery route, he was beginning to feel like total, you know what. He told me he probably picked up something at the local tire store while waiting for my car to get finished. He also told me he forgot to take his nutrition supplements that day. Now I know, and most of you know, that nutrition is so important. God wants us to be nourished. But we need to believe in the supernatural, super-nutritional things God has provided for us. So, when he got home with the chills and fever, I had the homemade soup ready, oils in the diffuser, and you better know it, look-it-up-girl had the negative emotion release answer waiting for him. I told him that he needed to choose to give the negative emotion of "believing the worst is happening" to God and replace it with the "best is happening." As I gave him bottled water, I asked him if he gave it to God, and he let me know that he had. I am happy to report, by morning, he let me know he was better. He still spent several days at home recovering, but it was not the terrible onset that appeared to be on its way through his body! Now, come on! No flu! And in hindsight, was it something worse?! How can that be? I have cut flu off at the pass with mega doses of nutrition, like very proactive aggressive nutrition, and was very successful. Flu and menopause are not really my styles, so I have never dealt with either one. But my husband choosing to give his negative emotions to God by way of his words, and there be a definite change eight hours later, tells me just to CHOOSE to let it go! He has seen it enough with me; I know he believes. Like probably most husbands with oils, emotional release, kale, they are like "this is all nice, honey, but please go and get me a beer and some Nyquil! Lol!

I have come to realize, believing smaller afflictions away gives you the faith to believe the bigger ailments away or maybe deter them all together! Flu is no joking matter, and I don't blame any mom that takes their baby to get a dose of something to minimize the awful effects. But when an opportunity to use emotional release presents itself, why not give it a try. As you hop in the car to head out to the doctor, try doing the verbal exchange, and see how you feel when you get to the office. How many times have we made the appointment and then suddenly feel better, like we know that things are in good hands? I always feel like my car runs smoother after I go to the carwash. Crazy, I know. Does anybody else have this experience? Perspective is a powerful cocktail we give our brain that eventually trickles down to our bodies. There are studies by the hundreds that prove a placebo is highly effective. It's kind of like the doctors administer a sweet little pill that causes hope to rise! Oh, my word, hope, not dope!

Chapter 10

The Gift Long Story Less Long

"It is encouraging to see the progress for something that can be so elusive! Pull the junk out of the obscure, invisible trunk and nail it to a piece of paper and watch your life change."

Whenever I am landscaping or tending my own garden at home, often, I will prick my finger on a thorn. I remember one time on a landscaping job, I had a Canary Palm thorn puncture my hand and break off. The x-ray didn't show it, but about three days later, it began to make its way out the middle of the back of my hand. Oddly enough, this was the day before Good Friday. You can always find me sprucing up a yard around this time of year, so I am continually reflecting on what Christ did for us on the Cross too. But a thorn coming out of the back of my hand; this was a little much. Whenever I have the unfortunate experience of a thorn getting me, I immediately wince and then think about what Jesus did. That was a whole lot of trouble to go through for me. I simply cannot wrap my head around it. Why on earth would He do all that for me? It's unimaginable, but I am so thankful that He saved me from that pain. And He has been taking my pain regularly as I give him the emotions that are afflicting my health. I would stop telling the world, but I cannot. Let me explain.

The S.H.I.T. is for real *meaning Ship High in Transit*

As I began to let my family and friends know the title of this book, I got some interesting feedback, as you can imagine. Some were like, "WHAT?!" Others were like, "Right on, Sister!" You would not believe the dot coms I now own as I tried to see if maybe something else would work for the title. I won't go into a long speech about how sometimes God makes you so very unique and then gives you radical grace to live out your calling, but there it is. Some of my friends and family let me know I could probably give it a much better title, and like me, I started coming up with a suitable alternative. I will say the best and most awesome title that did not end up in this book is one my dad clued me on. He's an avid "no swear words" kind of guy. And I think the funniest thing he says for an explicative is, "Well kiss Old Rose!" So, when I sat him down and told him the name, he immediately began to say to me one of the stories about how this provocative word came to be. He explained when Ships carried manure, they had the unfortunate discovery that the buildup of methane in the belly of the ship caused explosions, they came up with S.H.I.T., Ship High In Transit or Stow High in Transit. Of course, I totally love the "ship" one better! I just laughed and laughed, and I'm still laughing! I told him that it reminded me of handing your crap emotions up to God. I thought he would faint. So, to honor dad and the historic "Ship High In Transit," I have lovingly thrown that out as the title of this book.

I really have no idea of the date, but I can tell you it was a partly cloudy day, my favorite, and it was around eleven in the morning. I was cleaning and working around the house and truly relaxed. And then, out of nowhere, I have this pain in my right big toe. I had this same pain a few weeks before. It was excruciating, but it was gone after about twenty seconds. I didn't think of it or the emotional release for it again. It was gone. Then suddenly, it was back this day. Not only was it back, but it was also worse and not going away. It felt like an icepick was going through my right big toe! Thoughts went racing through my mind, and I, "Look-It-Up Girl," was thinking, how I could possibly see emotional release this away! As a matter of fact, I thought about how rude and terrible and full of it I was to tell people that they could use this to rid themselves of sickness and pain. The pain was horrible! So, I began my monologue to God, through the ceiling, and it went something like this. "Oh God, this hurts so bad I cannot imagine that I could emotionally release this away! But it hurts so bad!" All the while, I am thinking, *I can't believe I tell people to do this all the time!* "But, Lord, if I give my negative emotion to You, and this pain goes away, I will never stop telling people about this!" Having read enough reference books on the subject, and also piecing together very quickly in my mind the things that had been causing me fear, I spoke these words. "I'm guessing for my right toe on my right foot; I need to give You my fear of moving forward in business and life! And like BOOM, the pain vanished, instantly as I spoke those words, then exclaimed, the sh*t is for real!!! I began very thankfully to praise God. And next, the thought of shouting it from the rooftop came to my mind. So welcome to my rooftop! I have sat next to total strangers and talked to them about this. Amazingly, people do receive it! Sometimes the symptoms are so obvious they are shocked that you have some insight into what they are thinking. But the truth is it is displayed a lot of times on their bodies. In the back of this book, I will put some great resources if you want to begin to "look it up." Some of the narratives are compelling; some of them I throw out the window because they do not line up with my own beliefs, but the references to find out what emotions are causing your dis-ease, I have found to be most helpful. So, when I say look it up, this could give you a head start.

The Stuff that Hits the Fan *is for Real!*

The next chapter may be filled with information that you believe with all your heart, or for some, it may be a roller coaster ride of skepticism. But these are a few of the miracles of emotional release that I want to share; a few tributes to the amazing way God made our bodies to work. It really is a Gift!

One of my good friends called me one day and began to tell me about the miserable pain in her knee. She had seen our other friend online talking about the pain in her knee as well and its emotional tie to her daughter getting married. This friend's daughter was also getting married, and she called me right away to find out about the essential oil for that kind of emotion. It was funny, but when I told my mom this story, she recalled having knee pain before one of my sister's weddings. They really should call it Mother-of-the-Bride knee! We knew the oil blend called Present Time was the one to use. I let her know I would get it for her, but that we should do the emotional work right then and there on the phone so she could feel better right away. She agreed, and we began. I pulled up the emotions from my reference materials that corresponded with her aching knee, and we talked them out together. I said the sentences of releasing to God, and she repeated each, then I said the opposite or a Scripture to replace it, and she repeated. It was kind of funny. Just an unscripted set of sentences not well-spoken but heartfelt, then we were done. I asked her, "How does your knee feel now?" She answered immediately and excitedly, "Oh, wow! How does that work?" The pain was gone! I said, "Girl, God made us so miraculous!" Though I sent her the essential oil, the real gift was the immediate relief that came to her. This particular friend is always ready and willing to look at her emotions and hand them over to God! I love it because her results are also just as sudden!

I was an emotional eater for the longest time who would wake up in the middle of the night and chow down. I would appear to be awake and was but had no will power at all to stop myself. One morning when I woke up and realized that the stove was left on all night after I cooked peanut butter toast right on one of the gas burners, I made a doctor's appointment! I needed to see if I could get to the bottom of the issue since it was getting dangerous for our house and my waistline! So, after letting the doctor know my situation, she prescribed a diet pill for one month to take that would reset my schedule for eating. And even though the pill made me want to rip my husband's head off daily, I took it, and after a couple of weeks, the night eating ended. However, it came back about two years later. So, I got to the emotional root of why I was emotional eating in the middle of the night. After I gave the emotion to God and replaced it, I never experienced the night eating again! The emotions for hunger and weight are all interconnected in my experience. I finally realized after embarking on my feelings journey that my night eating was one hundred percent emotional!

When the *Feelings Buried Alive* book charts became available in app form, it was an amazing new world of instant healing information available to me. Which meant I didn't have to look in a book and flip back and forth to find answers for myself and others. I could open the app! I adapted the app to my style of emotional release! Let's face it, that exchange was between God and me. I would lay down at night and admittedly diagnose my family and friends. I did so as if I was the Nancy Drew of emotional health. Bev was frequently reminding me of the fact that you could not say what another person's negative emotions were or are. I knew that, but guessing was kind of interesting to me. I think in part because of my desire to be set free and see others set free and partly my desire to see if the symptoms and what I thought their issues were would be a match. Healing and transformation are my super-powers and my kryptonite! Analyzing addiction, remember. And my feeling responsible for encouraging, all the time can, in actuality, be a negative emotion if not kept in check. I bet you can never guess what it affects! Bingo! It affects your abdominal area. Encouragement is valuable, but being responsible for the outcome is where we need to draw the line when it comes to that. It's not easy to draw and is a line that is sometimes a great work of art when you master it.

Two years ago, during a trip to Tennessee, I met a woman at a Bible study in our friend's home. This sweet woman, that very day was put on a kidney transplant list I found out as we visited. Of course, you know, with my obnoxious self, I began to tell her that there were negative emotions that could affect the health of her kidney. She let me know that she felt several of the feelings, and then I asked her if she was ready to let them go. She said yes, and I led her through the releasing and replacing one by one. Then when we were all done, I prayed. Simple, right? Well, ten days later, her husband sends out a group text and lets us know that they found a match for her transplant, which was a miracle. My sweet new friend was texting me like two days later doing amazing, and she recovered miraculously! To this day, she is doing great! So, you know my brain says her new kidney will not have to deal with the old emotions from pre-release and replace!

Incontinence is a sign of a person being wary of controlling emotions, overflowing emotions, guilty of not being loyal to yourself. So, incontinence is often coupled with the various emotions that have to do with control—suffering from this until I took it out with emotional release. The relief that came was undeniable, and it cleared up immediately! When I had a sudden onset, I looked it up again. Done! So, there is always what you might call the rational thought that comes first. Or maybe you will suffer from an ailment without even thinking about it having an emotional root. But as you put this into practice, you will begin to change your thought patterns. Like these, "I guess I just have to live with this," or "I guess I need to have that procedure or medication."

Does this sound familiar? When I jumped on the UPS truck to help my driver husband at Christmas time, it provided me with endless opportunities to overcome physical ailments and limitations. Can you say, bladder failure?! So, this is where stopping to consider what you are thinking about helps. Imagine working with your husband on his very intense delivery job in your late forties, surrounded by the people that you go to luncheons with normally—all the while in the hot Texas Christmas heat. And the crappy plywood seat, jumping up and down, and in and out of a big truck, over and over again, would logically seem to be the reason for a sudden onset of incontinence and tailbone trauma. I would whine and fuss and ask him every day if I was being punked! Like what on earth was I thinking! And what on earth was he thinking! Well, I believe, later when it was all over, and I was like in great shape physically, I had my answer! And yes, we are still married! But later, I found out that the symptoms that I began to suffer with, the incontinence and bonus tailbone pain, did not originate with the crappy jump seat or my jumping in and out of the truck. When I fessed up to Beverly, while in Australia, and five weeks of grinning and bearing the awful tailbone pain and other symptoms, she let me know that there was no way with my healthy habits I could have anything grave going on in my body. She told me that she gathered it was a financial worry and that I needed to put an essential oil on my tailbone and give my financial worry to God! She knew me well enough and was spot on with her analysis! Well, seriously, I wish I would have fessed up BEFORE we flew to Australia! After I followed her unusual prescription that wiped out every terrible symptom, I was having for the prior six months, and I had a ball on our twenty-three-hour flight back home! To this day, I have never experienced those things again!

Fear *Aggression*

Many times, in my life, I have wondered why people do the things they do. Haven't we all? The question that gets me most often is, "Why they do the mean things they do?" Remembering back to earlier years, I know I brought that question up in the minds of family, friends, and total strangers on numerous occasions. In my behavior work with dogs and their pet parents, I can see many parallels. I spent a lot of years as a RED Zone girl, so I recognize it with ease. I do not believe any of us are born pissed off. Well, my oldest son has a newborn picture that made us often wonder. Kidding, of course, but the photographer had one heck of a bright light on him for that picture, and I don't think my son was ready for his close-up that day. He is the only one that I stayed in the hospital long enough to get the newborn picture, and it was before we all carried around our home telephone and photography studio in our purse or pocket, so it is the only one we have to show off. But I digress. Fear is just about the only thing I can think of that could make a loving person lash out at the nicest of people.

I remember Pastor Jesse Duplantis, say the funniest yet profound words. "Faith is God's way of saying, "Have a nice day!" That is the most challenging truth there is to follow in my personal experience. Letting go of what is troubling you is the answer. Giving it to God and making it His problem and responsibility is the key. Wading through the real-life work of it all can be a trial. But putting your head and heart in the right place on the matter can help alleviate the toll that that stress will take on your body. I have known several people, over the years, that have had multiple trips to the ER for what they believed was a heart attack. Talk about a hellacious false alarm. Everyone is always happy to find out they are not having a heart attack, but what a lot of bull to go through for something false. The diagnosis is always stress and anxiety. Yes, your heart races, but it is your emotions doing a number on your body! A couple of years ago, a friend invited me to a self-improvement, networking type event. I sat by a man where a chair was pulled out because I was late for the meeting. I am rarely late and almost always ridiculously early to things. The speaker asked us to share with each other what we needed improvement on in our personal and business lives; I turned and began to talk with my neighbor to the left. This sweet man that I was seated next to said he was, pretty much, an introvert and did not like to deal with drama. He said that he was working on having more patience with people. He also let me know that he was working on patience to keep his heart in good health as he had a decision to make on a recommended heart surgery. I immediately began asking him some very personal questions about how he felt, because, well, you know me. At first, he answered, "Not really." As the speaker began to start back on his topic, I looked up the emotions on my *Healing Feelings* app and passed the phone over to him. I mean, I am, after all, "Look it Up Girl!" I whispered that it could be one or some or none, and he began to give a nervous giggle. And then he whispered back to me that he felt every single one of the emotions mentioned on the list. After a moment of contemplation, he asked, "So this emotional stress is causing issues in my heart?" I told him I believed so and quickly and quietly let him know how to "release and replace." I then encouraged him that whatever he decided surgery-wise, he was going to be ok. At the break of the class, the gentleman and I headed out early to go on our ways. My good friend that invited me to the class walked me out, and I let her know that she placed me next to a lovely gentleman that I had the most interesting God appointed conversation with, I believed. She let me know that the friend that invited him had told her earlier that he did not believe in God. A thought occurred to me later that God had been the One to sit me next to that sweet gentleman to tell him the most seemingly strange information about emotions and his heart condition. I believe that with all my *heart*!

Failures *into Victories*

I have had so much fun typing as I write this book. The writer character in my most favorite movie, "You've Got Mail," Frank Nebaski, is so full of himself and so in love with his typewriter! I think I completely identify with him as I carry on clicking away at this laptop. In middle school, I began my typing class trials, and it was an absolute disaster of an attempt. It was one thing to have awful grades in math, but typing too! Now, come on! It was a terrible feeling, a bit like when I tried to do aerobics. No Fun! But now I feel a total sense of victory as I type away in these early hours.

Failure only has the power to cripple you if you let it. And believe me, I let it do just that for years. That is what happens, though, when you are a constant risk-taker. It is built into our DNA, some of us, and we just cannot help it. So why would failure break a risk-taker down so bad? I don't have an answer for that. I wish I did! I do know it is something that you, as you get back up again, can give to God and move on. I am always pitching the possible and re-strategizing my plans for my brain's sake; seeing your ability to jump back up as actual victory is a healthy habit for sure. In my very first emotional release class, I discovered a lot about this failure stuff and how I was not dealing with it at all. In our class, we looked up an emotion or an ailment and found the emotion to do the self-releasing exercise. We looked through the reference books to begin our detective work. I was prepared to pick "abandonment," as we were told, it is a common emotion for people, especially if you were taken from your mother in the hospital for any length of time. I have seen these issues also working at the animal shelter. So, I picked this emotion and decided it was an easy one to figure out for this exercise—lavender on the hip alarm points and the releasing verbiage to quote.

Easy right!? As I looked through the book, helping my classmates find their emotions and alarm points in the book, the word "failure" jumped off the page and grabbed me by the face with both hands. I didn't know words in a book could do that, but they sure can! I gasped and noted that the oil for this emotion is Peppermint! Well, call me Peppermint Patty because the day before, I saw another classmate open her mouth and pour in some Peppermint, so I decided to do the same. I wasn't even sure why I did that to tell you the truth. It can cause you to gasp when you see an emotion that resonates with you. It is a common occurrence. I guess that is why they call it an "aha" moment. So, this failure business is for real. I didn't even know that it was like a thing with me. I should've though, when earlier, after a ten-question quiz at the end of the Chemistry class on the day before, I had a freak-out. The quiz was not for credit and even had a fun question in it to make the test seem light-hearted. As the true or false answers came to light, I realized that I answered each question on the line below it! So, they were all wrong. After all the answers were read aloud, I stood up, very pissed off, and exited the room.

The next day as we did the self-releasing work in groups, I let my new besties know that I was feeling the weight of that test on me the day before. They let me know they were all wondering what happened to me and my happy demeanor. They were like, what? I told them I needed to drink the entire bottle of Peppermint next time, LOL! Funny, but in my work at the shelter where often, I use Peppermint to redirect a dog through their sense of smell, it does another fantastic thing as it helps the dogs. It lifts the spirits of my fellow SPCA human friends that deal with challenging situations regularly. Shelter work of any kind is rough! The peppermint, I would even venture to say, helps these dogs that have ended up at the shelter for one reason or another.

Can dogs have feelings of failure, and can peppermint do more than just redirect their nose, but help them to overcome feelings of failure? I can't prove it, but I just bet it does!

Less of Me *a lesson in getting over yourself!*

Recently, I was telling one of my good friends that I had been dealing with sore bones and muscles, a pain I had not experienced in quite a while. And this is" haven't shaved my legs," truth here! You can even write a book on this topic and still have significant issues pop up that need to be addressed. To be exact, not since I had started digging in on issues about jealousy and anger and so on. Jealousy, by the way, I call my stupid negative emotion. I am so blessed. We are all so blessed, and when I see someone else living out my lifelong dream, I just go nuts with jealousy! It is the dumbest thing. Truly!!! I was going to be the next Martha Stewart!!! Lol. Well, thank you, Chip and Joanna Gaines! Lol! But seriously, you may think I am nuts, and no way am I healed. But I kid you not, this is an actual conversation that I have had with my friends. And they try to convince me that I can still be and do all of that if I want to. Crazy, is it not? I have to tell all of you that I could not be more thankful for Chip and Joanna Gaines. They are one fantastic couple, and I love all that they stand for. The trickle-down of their business is nothing short of epic, and they have turned home improvement into a movement. I can remember the day I watched Joanna Gaines give her testimony on YouTube. It was titled "The

Gathering," and as she spoke to my business broken heart and feelings of failure, I burst into tears and began to let all types of emotions flow. Who was this woman? I figured out quickly who she was. She and her husband were responsible for me trying to find out how the homebuilder I worked for could put "paneling," AKA "Ship Lap" in buyer's homes. While I was too overworked to even dream of watching Fixer-Upper, I was helping implement those elements inspired by them into their homes.

I can also remember the day that I watched Chip at a men's conference, and when they finished, they prayed for him. I prayed too! Crying, I prayed, and it was very emotional! And then Chip lets everyone know he wants to jump out in the crowd and body surf on their hands. So, tears turned to laughter! In any event, jealousy is the dumbest emotion there is to me. It is real, though, and must be dealt with whenever it rears its ugly head! Thankfulness is always the remedy! I can remember the day my husband had a situation with his job, and I found myself telling God that I was not in the least bit jealous of Chip and Joanna Gaines, and I was so thankful for my own life! I am still learning not to gaze over the proverbial fence to drool and stare at another's "Pinteresting," greener grass. I know God is doing amazing things in my life, and I am thankful for the territory HE has given me.

So back to the muscle-skeletal issue. I decided to dig in on the emotion and deal with it, which always leads me back to my core issues. I had never put the emotion "pride" or the word "ego" as the thing I needed to release. But suddenly, I had a revelation that I needed to give all of that pride to God. I would replace it with healthy confidence. I

67

had a situation where I was not thinking and butted in on a trainers class up at the animal shelter. He politely refused my help, and I was like, oh crap! I was wounded instantly and embarrassed that I had done something so rude. I intended to help but, hello, what was I thinking? After I left, I sent an apology through the coordinator of volunteers, and it all was just fine. But I needed to deal with myself on a deep emotional level. EGO! PRIDE! When I dug in early in the morning before I started my morning dog walking routine up at the shelter, I addressed it and released and replaced it. After this, a fantastic thing happened. I was alone almost all of the morning, just the big dogs and me. That morning I was able to handle them better and effectively get them to follow my lead with minimal pulling. What the heck? I know that emotions affect the dog at the end of your leash. I teach this nearly every day. Confidence is a handy and useful tool that is effective! So, clear out the pride and take in its place CONFIDENCE! I could see so clearly the difference between these dogs. It was the key to getting over myself and becoming much more effective!

I have been dealing with my weight for years, and I attribute most of my getting in shape to emotional release. Emotions were the reason that I would night eat. It was the reason I would eat my box of cookies and your box of cookies, too, then think about where I was going to get my next box of cookies. And I have done some pretty extreme diets to lose weight then not keep it off. But I know when I started dealing with the emotions and eating healthy, that is when results began sticking. The "sheltercise," as I call it, has been instrumental in taking me to the next level. Anytime I do an intense exercise, I notice all types of issues, mostly anger, humiliation, pride, to name a few, come to the surface. I am a very happy person and display delight frequently. But I can also openly admit that I am a work in progress. I confess that I carry negative junk and then figure out what the replacement is because I want to improve my health every day! And just let me say that I sometimes suck at controlling my emotions! Sometimes I can wear my passion on my sleeve!

I admit it because I have learned the value of understanding where you are in life. You know that thing; confessing to another that you have not shaved your legs in months may be way easier than telling others your negative emotions, but bearing one another's burdens makes the journey a less lonely one. Embarrassing at times, but you are not alone. And then there is a type of accountability that is created by confessing your negative emotions to one another. I am not saying write all of your junk in a published book or anything, which must be my epic strategic way to have maximum accountability! Welcome to my madness, lol! But seriously taking all of this and confiding in a person you can trust and even journaling it all out is an efficient way to do this modality. It is encouraging to see the progress for something that can be so elusive! Pull the junk out of the obscure, invisible trunk and nail it to a piece of paper and watch your life change.

So, besides giving up pride and taking on real healthy confidence, there is also a selfish thing. You figure that out, and how to give it to God, it is a great way to overcome, period! Less of ME! In life, I want to value myself, but I also want to get over myself! Less of Me! The weight issues, the jealousy issues, the anger issues, the selfishness, they have to go! It is like you take your flesh and all its fleshly tendencies and hand it up to God! No, woe is me! Less of me! For several years now, I have had a sign that is intended for a little girl's room, which hangs by my front door. It says, "Hello Little Lady," I bought it initially for my granddaughter that lived in our house with my son and daughter-in-law for a couple of years, but then I thought this was good for me to see every day. It encompassed all that I needed to believe or wanted to believe. Childlike faith, to be little in size, LESS of ME. Hello, little lady! This powerful thought is what I see as I leave the house every day! When I open the door to let puppies in and out, time after time, I see it! But it is not just the weight issue. Recently, I have been getting a powerful message about what that means on a deeper level! Less of ME! It is to let go of my "way of doing" it and all the emotional baggage attached. It is a goal I can fall short of for sure, but it is a beautiful balance where you partner with God and His restful and restorative journey

Chapter 11

Healed Right Before My Eyes

"Now you see it now you don't!"

At the beginning of this book, I mentioned the healing of flesh that I had immediately witnessed three times. And I have experienced other rapid healing of my flesh, not instant but miraculous just the same. Instant healing is something that your brain begins to question, and you are grateful when there are other witnesses to it. Healing flesh is so cool because it is something you can see with your eyes. Not that other instant miraculous healing isn't astounding; it's just that you get to see it happen.

My daughter was playing on the swing set at our local park one time. She could run like the wind and climb on everything like a ninja warrior. I can't remember exactly how old she was, but I know it was before she was too cool for the local park and specifically the swing set. As I sat near, on the park bench, and began to read Dodi Osteen's book on healing, she was playing so carefree not far away. Page after page, it held me captive until I stopped, and looking up, I witnessed Savannah drop from holding on to the top bar of the play structure. As she landed somehow, her little body folded up like an accordion, to where her chin hit the ground between her legs. As she jumped up from this leap-frog position, she began screaming. In shock, I gazed at the blood on her tongue in the shape of her top teeth. She ran to my arms, and as she did, I patted her on the back with a consoling gesture and exclaimed, "Oh honey, mouths heal really fast!" No sooner than I spoke these words, she was fussing at me, "Let me down, let me down!" I let her down but stopped her from running back to the swing set to give it another go so that I could look in her mouth. No blood, completely healed, is what I saw! How amazing was that! A healing conversation, proclamation, or whatever you would like to call it. Not even an official prayer. Some might even say it was the anointing coming off Miss Dodie's book, but in any event, it was totally miraculous!

On another occasion, a healing miracle happened as I sorted through roses that were being used for a Couple's Ministry at my church. I used to be extremely active as a church volunteer. I don't have a medium speed button, so my all or nothing attitude led me to be at a myriad of volunteer positions. I think my favorite by far was leading children's worship. But I digress. As we began working on the roses, one of the women in the group realized we had not prayed before we started working. That is like totally a thing at churches, and I have witnessed it warding off gossip and micro-managers, big time. She prayed that God would bless the work of our hands, etc. And then we got back to work.

Before long, we were finished and cleaning up the stems and leaves that were trimmed off the centerpieces. As I swooped up, yes, that is the proper use of the word swoop, at least in Texas it is! I swooped up a bundle of plant material, and a huge thorn sliced through my left thumb! In an instant, a large bead of blood came through the thin skin that I was always peeling off my thumbs. I gasped for air and then suddenly remembered the prayer! "Lord, I thank You that we prayed and asked You to bless the work of our hands. So, my thumb is healed!" As I said these words, I was placing my index finger over the wound. As I released it, I looked to see my thumb totally healed! So healed, in fact, that even the skin I had peeled off was entirely back! Seriously! No prayer and fasting, just matter-of-fact believing. I've had to repeat this account to myself through the years. There's an urge to think it was just my imagination, even if there was another witness.

That brings me to an incredibly awesome healing miracle that I talk about so often. It was just the coolest ever! I mean, miracles always are! Am I right? One afternoon sending my son off on an overnight church retreat, I saw a friend of mine and her daughter. They were dropping off her older girls, and she had her youngest held closely by her side with a small white cloth over her head. I noticed her daughter was calm and collected as they came closer. I also noticed that my friend was very pregnant. As we began to talk and catch up, it had been a while; I found out she was eight and a half months pregnant and that her sweet daughter with her had gashed her head on the play equipment at our children's school.

She pulled back the cloth, the sight of the hole in her head was in the shape of an eye and very deep. In the second before I winced and squinted my eyes, I saw several layers of flesh the injury had opened. I have never wanted to be a doctor, just play one on TV! Lol! We chatted for a few more minutes, and she let me know that while her other children were heading off to a retreat, she and this little one would be heading to the emergency room. They began to walk away, and I yelled, "Hey, wait up! Come here, little girl," I laid my hand on her head to pray. I thank You, Lord, that You died on the Cross and shed your blood so that eight and a half months pregnant women do not have to go to the ER. I thank You, Lord, that she is healed, and that they will look at it and not have to go to the ER! I thank You Lord, they will go home and have an enjoyable, relaxing evening together! Eloquent, I know!

The next day when we returned to pick up our children in the same spot we prayed, we met up again, and my heart was already filled with excitement because I knew! Her daughter was smiling, she was smiling, and I was smiling. She said it was healed! I asked, "Emergency room"? She said we turned the car around and went home! And now not a hair out of place! Not to be all "thorn in the side," but we looked all through that child's hair and could not find any evidence of the wound!!! God is so good!!! It was such a great feeling, so awesome! About one year later, I was walking to get my kiddos from school, and I saw my friend in the line of cars waiting. She rolled down her window, and we exchanged hellos. I began to ask her about her daughter's head; I didn't even get the question out before she said to me, "Not a hair out of place!" We laughed, and I told her, "Thank you!!!" As she drove away in the line, I rejoiced! It is so fun to remember and celebrate the miraculous.

As impressive as miracle healings are, and I am so thankful for them, there are other miracles to be told and miracles to be had by so many. Because God made our bodies to heal, He also made our bodies to signal us when we need to deal with things that are not good for our soul. It reminds me of the guy in that game, Operation. You know how things light up when you touch the side of the opening. Well, I think God made our bodies to light up and send a signal to us. Inflammation, small at first, then like a bonfire! I always want to take the emotion out when it is just a little flicker, and not when I am so full of inflammation; my body is sending up smoke signals. Other symptoms can scream out at us that can lead us to look for answers. Sometimes the doctor will tell you it is stress-related, and other times they will simply tell you that all your tests are negative, and they can find nothing wrong with you. Below is a list of just a few of the most amazing miraculous healings that I have personally experienced. I have seen many other accounts in those who have grabbed hold of this concept and used it. These are just a few of my own miracle healings with their associated emotions, and a few of my husband's;

Immobilizing pain in my left shoulder blade – Overwhelmed
Pain in my tailbone and rectal bleeding – Financial worry
Thyroid diagnosed and medicated for two years – Humiliation
Intense almost crippling hip pain – Deep sorrow and grief, unforgiveness of self
Incontinence – emotionally weary, duh!
Joint pain – Anger

Hunger – Longing for love

Fat – Need for protection

Allergies – Someone or something is getting on your nerves

Gums and teeth - unworthy

Chronic car sickness – CONTROL, even as a child

Look for indications from your own body. There are the references you can go to; *Heal Your Body* and such. But in time, if you use emotional release regularly for your health, you will almost intuitively know what the emotion is. I have an incredible memory, and after a while, I begin to think about the memorized reference charts. Truthfully, there is a core set of emotions that all the other feelings can stem from, based on, or related too. It sounds like a family tree of yuck!

My right foot that I am always working on the emotions for is like a textbook scenario! I have come to believe that those Israelites that did not make it into the Promised Land most likely had problems with their right foot or right big toe! I am always talking about the places I will not step one toe into ever. The moving forward thing is a life's work for sure. Having difficulty moving forward into my destiny and thinking about many small details is a constant battle for me. Talk about going toe to toe on an issue. But it gets better all the time, and when I get a right foot big toe flare-up, I know exactly what to release and replace.

Now you feel it; now you don't! Just like forgiveness that we don't always think is true right away, so I believe it is with our emotions! No abracadabra here! In an interview years ago, Martha Stewart was asked about getting sick. She answered, "I'm never sick. I try never to be sick. Why get sick? It's a waste of time." Her words resonated with me so strongly! "Yes," I thought! "Seriously, what is the point of that?" Mind over matter and basically refusing the condition of sick.

My husband and I both have ignored injuries on many occasions. And like the determined maniacs we were, we continued with activities that our injury should have prevented us from doing. I know my ankle healed funny because I refused to let falling off a ladder keep me from leading children's worship. Sprained ankle and all, I was jumping up and down at church a couple of hours after the accident. I remember painting the side of my house years ago, and my ladder fell over. The paint flew up in the air and landed on my head. It happened just as if I was in a movie or something, which was not what I wanted to be my cinematic debut. So, I snuck inside my house, hoping the neighbors did not see me. I needed to get to my church and carry out my volunteer duties, and this dumb injury was not stopping me. I literally threw some natural concoction on it and refused to acknowledge the pain. Radical oiler and radical volunteer, I was. The injury did not have the power to keep me down. Once my husband injured and broke the bones of his hand in a very peculiar place between his fingers. He did this skateboarding of all things. He was not injured on the job, so that was another overwhelming consequence of having fun and being a package handler for employment. You cannot afford to be injured off the job or really on the job for that matter. It all sucks financially. But somehow, this man was back to work in a matter of days!

Another truly miraculous healing happened after an injury catching a fly ball at a softball game then misjudging where the fence was. He destroyed his rotator cuff, tore his bicep, and a couple of other problems were noted on his MRI. We spent nearly every day, hopeful and depressed all at the same time. On one particular Sunday, a few days after the MRI, we packed up the kids and drove to church. As I write this, I can feel the crap feelings of it all try to wash over me again! Maybe there is more releasing and replacing I need to do here. By the way, writing, what a gift! Journal your body the Good News! Anyway, I remember it, and it was no fun! So, there we were at church, and basically, grinning and bearing it.

The preacher started talking about worship and healing, then discussed some of the epic-level miracles he had experienced. He said there was healing in worship. It was beautiful! Back then, Ron and I were not fans of standing, hands raised while worshiping. We were more like the type to sit and read every square inch of the bulletin and avoid at all costs any display of veneration. But this day, the preacher told us to stand to our feet and raise our hands in thanksgiving to God. In my mind, I was like, "Well, you are not the boss of me! And, by the way, I am just getting to the good part of this bulletin, mister!" And then suddenly, my very not charismatic, down to earth, dry sense of humor, Ron, jumps to his feet and raises both of his hands full on above his head! You know, like the thing you cannot possibly do when you have the type of injuries he had to his arm, that we were yet to now he had. Remember, we were still waiting on the results of the MRI.

This man stood up. And I stood up. As we did, hands raised, his raised higher than mine, I was having trouble even believing what I was seeing. When the service was over, we grabbed the kids and headed to the car. I turned to him, walking through the parking lot, and said, "Honey, do you think we just got a miracle?" He leaned sideways without looking at me and said, "Let's not talk about it and just get in the car." On a side note, quite often, when a seriously real miracle of God happens, I've noted, people do not want to discuss it right then; they want to wait to get in the car or go home to discuss it. It's like this weird phenomenon that happens after the most amazing things. After church, we went to my sweet in-law's house for lunch like we did most Sundays. As we walked to the door to go in, a giant step ladder weighing about twenty-five to thirty pounds sat next to the door. In one fell swoop, Ron picks it up and lifts it over his head, injured arm fully extended to heaven! Miracle confirmed! I jumped up and down, and he remained as calm as can be, as always!

The next day, a Monday, he left the house to head out surfing. I can't remember if I went with him or not. Surfing, where you need to paddle constantly, and most times extend your arm out as part of the activity. A few days later, he went to the doctor for his MRI results. Ron sat quietly as the doctor held up his results and began to show him the four places his arm was severely damaged and let him know that he needed surgery. He began to explain to Ron that the recovery time would be a minimum of six months out of work. At that point, Ron jumped up off the exam table and began to move his arm in a large circular motion exclaiming, "Dude, I am fine! I went surfing this past week! Can you write me a note to go back to work?" Jaw dropped, and in total shock, the doctor let him know that based on his MRI, he needed surgery. But based on what he saw just then, he would go ahead and write him a note to go back to work! To this day, Ron still has a bicep that is only attached at one end. Ron's miracle. It is like a memorial stone that his boss has even told other drivers to look at and stop their whining about their ailments. It is the cutest, funniest, Popeye-Esque muscle and is a reminder to us of what God does!

Parenting *the Greatest balancing act ever!*

My son Donovan, our middle child, came onto the scene at ten pounds two ounces. We did not find out if he was a boy or a girl before birth. I, my entire pregnancy, kept calling him little sister to his big brother, Ron. So much so that after he was born, little Ron called his little brother, sister, for about a week! He is the child that was born after my mother acquired her excellent videography skills and a fancy video camera. This woman could fade in and out and set up intriguing visual shots like a pro! I told her as I put on my lipstick at my house, getting ready to leave to go to the hospital after my water broke, "Do not film this baby coming out of my body!" When the doctor or nurse suggested the mirror to watch, I was like, "Are you kidding me"? I had not wanted to see myself in a mirror for nine whole months. Why in the "bleepola," would I want to see that now? Some people are all ecstatic about it, but I will pass. Thank you. So, there we were at the hospital, and I made sure my mom understood my orders. She said she did. LIES! When push came to shove, literally, a very sentimental, well-meaning, STUPID nurse talked my mother into filming this 10 lb. 2 oz. baby coming out, and BONUS, one seriously awful hemorrhoid in view! As I write this book, I am releasing and replacing it all right now, lol! Not!

The only people to watch this video after the birth was one of my childhood friends and my sweet grandfather! I am not sure exactly how Grandpa got a hold of that video at my mom's house one Easter gathering, but he watched it upstairs in the game room and came down and declared that it was just like watching a National Geographic show! What a review on my cinematic debut! Needless to say, I confiscated the videotape and lost it somewhere forever. And maybe, God willing, it will never surface until all the VHS machines are wiped off the face of the planet! And the only person in the world that this video would have been maybe a good memory for would have been my son. Oh, wait, NO!

I don't know about all ya'll, but NO indeed. I heard several years later that you are not allowed to film in a regular hospital. Whether it was true or not, I figured it was a malpractice thing. I thought it would have been a good thing for me back then! And the entire labor time, we kept hearing things being knocked over off tables. Even so, I am happy they caught the baby when HE arrived! So, while my mom was breaking new cinematic ground, and I was being told that my new baby was a giant baby boy and not a wee tiny baby sister, I spoke out these words in a less than cinematic way. "It is?" The video recorded the disappointed sound in my voice. My son was adorable, and after I caught my snap, drugs scaled back, sutures finished up, and I held him in my arms, and my sweet Donovan became the child I would baby and try to never, ever make him feel like he was a middle child. I did this even when I was unaware that I was going to have another child.

When I found out my third baby was a girl, I had to load on the adoration to compensate for the guilt over my ecstatic joy. By the way, my son Donovan was also born on a Wednesday. Good Lord! My other two amazing kids let me know, for years, they knew Donovan was my favorite. I told them I could not love any of them more than the other, but that his behavior was much preferred. He asked me if I needed help with the groceries and told me when I looked pretty. He was easily corrected and put himself to bed when the sun went down! I mean, come on! I told them I would give my life for all of you, but his behavior, what's not to love?

But all kidding aside, my point is to show you how one small moment in time and how you feel can change your behavior for a lifetime. As I said earlier, I know plenty of people that are trying to live a life that is good and right and beat themselves up for falling short. Moms are in this category; I think most of all. My good friend and I are always discussing it! Oh, my goodness M.O.M., Mine Or Mine. The fault and the guilt! Let's think about this! I will say that now that I have grandchildren, they are my new favorites! Now, I think things like; God doesn't love us like a Father; HE loves us like a Grandfather.

Well, let's face it. God is the grandest Father ever! I had a friend tell me once you will never know until you have your own grandchildren, what it feels like, and you just can't explain it. Well, of course, in my over-analytical brain, I think, "challenge accepted," and figured out how to explain why we feel about them the way we do! I believe it's like the most incredible art that your children have ever made, and God helped them create this little masterpiece! If I had known, back in that delivery room, making my cinematic debut, I would have been a more balanced parent, and maybe they would have all felt like favorites. Letting all that go, though, is crucial to be the best me I can be right now for my family. And, for that, I am so grateful.

TMI *Just say NO to the Drama!*

It is a well-known fact in my family that I have this weird way of watching a movie or program that I have recorded or bought on DVD repeatedly and obsessively. Like who even does that anymore? I would stop what I was doing and ask my husband a question or do something to get his attention. Ron would be so funny and tell me, "Wait, I haven't heard this part of the movie before." We played the movie so many times we could recite it word for word! I really wouldn't watch the movie, necessarily, but have it running while I cleaned house or worked on a project—kind of like an early HGTV with a plot. I love movies with beautiful sets and scenery. I could play the film in my photographic memory, so I didn't need the screen. And the music of Home Alone, well what is not to love. That movie made us laugh as a family so hard; it was medicine to me. Of course, when I played it for the two-hundredth time, the fun wore off, but the visuals as I passed by the TV and the awesome Christmas music were very soothing to me. It reminded me of good times with my brood. And let's face it, the McAlister's were nuts like our family! I loved it!

In my severe "mom on overload" days, the kids and I celebrated what was affectionately named *Summer Denial Days*. I would put on the Home Alone DVD, close all the drapes, crank down the a/c and ignore the Texas heat! We would eat fun snacks and have wintery meals and live it up! I was nuts!!! I also remember opening the kitchen window so that I was aware of my behavior with my kids. I didn't want to run with all my "overloaded" urges to yell at them, so opening the window was a useful coping tool, no good for the insane electric bill, but good for my mom's consciousness. Do you see how miraculous it is that my kiddos survived? In those days, I did everything I could to keep wonderful visuals in front of me. I never turned on the news. The news was not in your face twenty-four-seven, but when we could afford to have cable, I quickly learned that I could not turn on CNN because it made me want to go out and kick some ass and take on all the injustices in the world. Guarding my mind was something that I learned to do like a Navy Seal. I would guard my mind against external news and unpleasant visuals, but I was not very good at controlling the negative narrative that existed in my head. I didn't know how to. One day the, take every thought captive verse came onto my radar, and I began to do that obsessively. My Bible studies as a child told me that, but it came alive in later years when I realized what a war zone my head had become. Now, at this moment in history, the battle to keep your mind free of new visuals, sound bites, and bad news is like never before! I still do not watch the news, not any of it. And though I am healed and whole now, I refuse to participate in the madness of it all.

I remember growing up on the show *Days of Our Lives*. When I hear the intro sound bites for the show, it is oddly comforting. It reminds me of a time when my lunch was made for me, and I played with my toys a lot. It also causes memories of naptime. The show that came on before *Days of Our Lives*, I think, was *As the World Turns*. If I heard that musical intro today, it would totally remind me of thinking how stupid naps were, lol! But as soft and melodic as the introduction was and is, in later years, I remember seeing one of the main characters on *Days* become possessed by the devil, and she began levitating! I thought to myself, "I think I am way too intelligent for this," and that ended my viewing of soaps for good! Hello, daytime drama, and finally, good riddance to daytime drama! We didn't need it! With all our family's craziness, we had a cottage industry of homemade drama!

These days there is a program running all the time all around us! I can remember telling my daughter, Savannah, that she could not text while we were riding in the car together. I told her that was our time together, and her friends were not allowed to jump into our mother-daughter realm by way of her flip phone. So funny to me now. Who did I think I was messing with anyway? I wonder if I would have held out longer on the whole kids and cell phone thing if I would have known. So, it's no secret that the more connected we are "virtually," the less we are actually connected! And what about the value of ACTUAL! Without a doubt, you can reach far and wide on social media. But, my serious old-fashioned self believes that showing up FOR REAL can reach a massive amount of people with no harmful side effects.

And knowledge, true or false, can be created online with ease today. Depending on the speed of your internet, WIFI, or data plan, you can have the info in seconds. I lovingly call this ability "The Tower of Google"! Information at your fingertips day in and day out is convenient, but is it healthy? Talk about TMI! All this is to say, just like the Hallmark movies filled with cupcakes and candy, I will never eat again, and romances my husband and I will never have, the soaps and news were filled with too much drama! And fast forward to this modern overload of drama, well, I have committed to saying NO! I resist the daily watching of news, as not to cause flu-like symptoms in my body! I don't think we were created to ingest information the way we do. I do not want a daily dose of drama that is spoon-fed to me and affects my behavior.

There are so many good things in this world to focus on today. And if you can't manage to find any, then make some goodness! I want to make progress; not collect new negative emotions daily. Putting on your "God armor" and giving it your all is a simple yet hard to remember habit. Needing to be reminded, for me, is day-to-day. I could be "Mary Sunshine" and then complain like the "Grinch" in the next breath! So, when my best attitude habit falls through, I use my backup habit that is to apologize. If I think about the negative stress I need to clear out of my mind, body, and life, why on earth would I want to create that for someone else to deal with in their being as well. It's a powerful thought.

I am not saying you never have to address situations where there is not agreement and problem solving needed among one another. I am talking complaining and fussing at someone when we are unhappy about something. If I envision that my negative words are like blobs of slime, and what happens when I direct them at someone or even myself, then that paints a most potent visual for the negativity! I do not want to go around sliming innocent folks! And I do not want to walk around sliming myself with negative self-talk. And that also goes for a situation that is not cleared up quickly. Do not let that negative situation slime you! If we remember in these situations to think happy thoughts, we can use those thoughts as our "slime deflectors"! I can remind myself of everything that God says about me. This very morning when I realized I read one of my due dates wrong on a bill and discovered that I am four days late in paying it, I started to play a very negative tape over and over in my mind. I began to think of a late charge, and so on. So, I stop myself from doing that. I tell myself to let it go! I am not an idiot, a slacker, or forgetful. Don't allow your whole day to get derailed by negative self-talk. It is such a waste of a day and is too much like a daytime drama! Decide that if your day is going to be dramatic, it is going to be an epic and fantastic drama that has everybody crying happy tears at the end!

Chapter 12

Go Epic or Go Home

"The battle is real, but the answers are real too."

Speaking of epic, check this out. I woke up from a dream this morning that was quite disturbing in the beginning, then had a fantastic twist, and by the end, I discovered some interesting insights. I was house sitting in a vast mansion, a very wealthy person's place, and it was beautiful! All at once, there was a break-in by two guys who wanted me to open a safe. Somehow or another, I knew that the police were alerted and were on their way. Anyhow, I also knew that these bad guys were not really so bad and that this act was one of desperation. I cannot remember if the guys had a gun or not. Determined to talk them out of their plan was more my focus in this dream than anything else. I incessantly and insistently told them that this was no good for them. They needed to know there was nothing in this house that was worth destroying their lives over. One guy kept telling me that I didn't understand and that he needed to do this. In my dream, we kept hearing distant sirens that didn't seem to get closer; but warned of the pursuit.

As we entered a massive closet, by the way, I have been organizing a lot of closets lately as it is one of my side hustles. Lol! As we entered the closet, we began to debate. I wouldn't let up as I continued to sell the idea that he could let go of this plan and start a good life. At some point, we realized that there was a ticking noise in the closet. This very loud ticking began to drown out the sound of the sirens. Suddenly, the three of us realized that this closet had an explosive device that was going to go off. I wasn't sure if the device was supposed to protect the safe or if this homeowner had it as a protection from safecrackers.

Dreams are funny like that, but suddenly the guy that I had been debating with threw down his belongings and began to deactivate the bomb! As I crouched in the closet corner, the man transformed into a hero who was there to save the day. When the police arrived, I let them know that these men saved our lives and the house from harm. The guy let me know he had always wanted to do something useful with his skills, and he never saw a way.

Now all of this probably seems very idealistic and in real life would maybe start a serious debate, but hey, it was a dream. When I break this dream down, it becomes a compelling analogy, illustration, and learning experience for me. When I think about it, sometimes I am that bad guy in the dream—trying with all my might to make things work out my way, no matter who or how it affects others, including me! I'm thankful when God provided a way out for me, and miraculously orchestrated a way to take all my junk and drama and turn it around into my awesome destiny. Sometimes I am me, in the dream, trying to talk people into choosing the better option for their lives. Other times

I am the bomb, ready to slime everyone for the sake of protecting myself, what I want, and what I believe is right. And a lot of times, I am just the siren in the background going on and on! Upon waking from this dream, I became so happy about how it turned out and then promptly forgot it until I began to write.

Rewriting your story and keeping it clean from all the damaging thoughts. We have a way to rewrite it. We have a way to clear out the nemesis. We have a way to keep it safe from harm. The battle is real, but the answers are real too. As I read through this book, I have found so many thoughts that I feel as if I am reading it for the first time! One of my thoughts was, "I am real, I have real feelings, and they need to be released, not stuffed." My feelings matter, and they will become matter if I don't deal with them. We were given these bodies of frail flesh so that they could tell us when we have unresolved, buried issues of the heart. We need to work out our health with fear and trembling and give our unresolved feelings to God. That's a great exchange to see healing. Getting mad and getting over it will not do. Getting angry and "getting over it" is what it is all about. Relationship!

So, this next thought came to me on one of my editing mornings. This book is not called what it is called for nothing, so here goes.

How many of you are the robbers in the dream? How many of you want to keep your old junk, the way you have always "been," because you refuse to change? You refuse to heed the warning that the distant sirens are calling out. A bomb in your health could go off if you do not dig in and start unlocking all the negative that you have stored in your body! Maybe you are waiting for the Navy Seals to barge in and save you, when the truth is, you have had the power all along. When we hit heaven's door, what a release and replace that will be, but I say, put all of that aside for now, and let's get our healing right now! Then let's take up our sick beds and go and let's set some other captives free!!!

Chapter 13

Forecast Awesome

"God's promises for us did not change from yesterday
to today or last year to this year."

As I bring this book to a close, I realize there are so many unique insights I have discovered in writing this book. It has blessed me in ways that I will forever be grateful for the rest of my life. My last name Schreiber, as I mentioned early on, means *writer* as in pencil pusher. At the first revelation of its meaning, I will admit it was a shocker. My name does not mean *author*. But as I began to mull it over, and reflect on all of the "pencil-pushing" with God, morning after morning, I am so glad I gave my writing and my name to God! I would rather be His *scriber* any day than an author on my own! A release and replace of revelation that has been both amazing and humbling.

So, I have been saying this lately, and it cracks my bestie Bev and me up. Hey! Why don't we just go ahead and believe the Bible?! Sometimes the delivery of Good News is so awkward that it seems like maybe we cannot say a word. I get it, and there have been times that I was called to hush up, but not many. The persecution that comes to those telling the Good News can most often come from our own head! Personal persecution! Decide to throw that out and become your own prophet for GOOD! Dig deep and find the promises of God! You might be thinking that this world we live in now seems all too "End Times-ish," where all is bleak. But I say, God's promises for us did not change from yesterday to today or last year to this year. Confess those promises of Good News, and give the devil a lousy day! You have nothing to lose by doing this and everything to gain! Those promises are the gifts that keep on giving! Confess your forecast and call it "Awesome"!

While writing this book and working at the local shelter, I have seen some genuinely incredible souls smile through and bless every living thing around them, even when stress is painfully high and, by the way, know the true meaning of "the shit is for real"! On my phone, I put the words "the awesome" after their names in my contacts; Jay the Awesome, Anne the Awesome, Dayna the Awesome, Rene the Awesome, Rebecca the Awesome, Sam the Awesome, Laura the Awesome, Anna Elise the Awesome, to name just a few. They are truly awesome, and their commitment is unwavering! I would ask them questions like, "What draws you to professions that have caregiving, nurturing aspect to them?" "How is it that you have a smile on your face, always, no matter how chaotic everything is around you?" All their answers have a common thread, LOVE. They love what they do, the animals, and to nurture and care. But the common thread through all of their answers, whether spoken or unspoken, is LOVE. It has blessed me so, and it is an illustration to me of how *love* is the greatest tool to overcome the difficulties of life. Loving the unlovable, loving when love is not returned, and loving because it is your default, is a special way to live life and overcome seemingly impossible circumstances. They are love with its sleeves rolled up! Their awesomeness has taught me that it changes the atmosphere around them!

No matter your position, there is a climate change that you can affect any day and every day! There is so much good in this world. And, there is so much more to be excited about than not. The pandemic mindset and viral infection mindset leaves much to be desired in the quality of modern-day. Ugliness and bitterness overshadowing the good and beautiful in life can be a root of emotion that spreads like a nasty weed on our society! So, when you see neighbors helping neighbors and everyone that is not vulnerable in body and mindset spreading good cheer in a gloomy hour, it is to me, the *good overcoming* that puts everyone in a healthier state. "Panic-demic" avengers, who, in a crisis, are willing to leave people, places, and things better than they found them, are a treasure. Who isn't made better by first responders of Good News? Let's decide to make "Goodness" go viral.

It is hard for me to remember sometimes, but we are called to be sweet! When I began this journey to scribe, I never realized that this world would transform into a very different place than it was when I started writing this book. For a transformation junkie, it is the mission field everywhere I look or go. As I sat to write this book, I have had a curious ailment clear up that I have had for about four years. This stupid rash! I have looked up every emotion that has had to do with the armpit area! Yes, armpit! There was no relief no matter what I did, and I have analyzed this rash and its corresponding emotions for the longest time to no avail. It made no sense. And I seriously have all those skin healing miracles in my past that I can reflect on. Funny that I am choosing to end my book on this subject matter, but hey, it is a labor of love, rashes, and all. As I have sat in my chair morning after morning, meeting God and His great love as I wrote, I have seen this rash begin to clear up. And when I started to speak Good News to those who are traumatized by recent events, the rash vanished altogether! What?!

Early one morning, as I looked up emotions for a dear friend, skin rash was one on the list. As I wrote it all up for her, I looked to type the last negative emotion of skin rash, and there it was. "Feeling frustrated at not being able to accomplish something." At the moment, my eyes landed on the words; I was overwhelmed. I realized the emotion that affected me for years, and its related ailment was gone. As I stood up and cupped my face into my hands, completely overcome with a feeling of overwhelming love and purpose, I got a vision of my swinging arms and the Lord taking His outstretched hand off my head saying, "Go get 'em, baby girl!" I believe that speaking what the Lord has put on your heart and walking in what you are meant to do will bring deliverance to your health, mind, body, and soul. I keep hearing over and over in my head, "Take up your sickbed and walk. Take up your sickbed and walk. Take up your sickbed and walk." Friend, I believe we must be willing to let go of past hurts and disappointments and the things that have no place in our lives. While we exchange them with a loving God for His goodness, I believe we will yank up that sickbed and run into the extraordinary and beautiful destiny He has for us.

If you are trying to release and you are not getting anywhere, there are a couple of things I have discovered of late that you can try. If there is a pain in your body and the release is not coming, you can think about someone else that you may be worried about in your heart and mind. And then think of how they are feeling and release and replace with those thoughts in mind. On several occasions, I have had to think about this. And when I thought about lifting up the emotions, I felt like they were feeling, I got immediate relief! Another trick up my sleeve is to take the concept of giving your pain a size and a color that I mentioned in an earlier chapter and put it on paper! Like art therapy! Draw it! Color it! You can write it out or illustrate it out!! As an artist, this is something I can relate to myself. When I was younger, I met a family that overcame a significant loss and tragedy with art therapy. The children painted their way to freedom. To me, it was so powerful. It is all a part of telling your body the good news. Let it go, and you will end up with a beautiful masterpiece of health!

About the Author

A self-described transformation junkie, Tracey has spent her life dedicated to changing the world around her and making it a better, more beautiful place for every living thing, whether in design, health, community outreach, or her philanthropic work. Passionate about the emotional connection to health and wellness, Tracey believes every person can live their best life if they take time to look deeper into the issues that surround their pain and sickness. Her wisdom and heart to teach and train has given her opportunities galore to see the remarkable results of bringing balance to our emotions and outlook on life.